LEARNING THROUGH MOVEMENT

Activities for the Preschool and Elementary Grades

SECOND EDITION

BETTY ROWEN

School of Education and Allied Professions
University of Miami

Teachers College, Columbia University
New York and London 1982

LIBRARY
COLLEGE OF ST. BENEDICT
St. Joseph. Minnesota 56374

Published by Teachers College Press, 1234 Amsterdam Avenue,
New York, New York 10027

Copyright © 1963, 1982 by Teachers College, Columbia University.

All rights reserved. No part of this publication may be reproduced or transmitted in any form or by any means, electronic or mechanical, including photocopy, or any information storage and retrieval system, without permission from the publisher.

Library of Congress Cataloging in Publication Data

Rowen, Betty.
  Learning through movement.

  Includes unacc. melodies.
  Bibliography: p. 99
  Includes index.
  1. Musico-callisthenics. I. Title.
MT948.R7 1982   372.13   82-3317
ISBN 0-8077-2720-2 (pbk.)   AACR2

Manufactured in the United States of America

87 86 85 84 83 82   1 2 3 4 5 6

LIBRARY

MT
948
.R7
1982

Contents

163614

7 ⁊❧ *Conclusion* 96

Acknowledgments

The material for the first edition of this book was gathered from my experiences as a classroom teacher in elementary school and nursery school, and as a dance teacher in community centers and private schools. The additional material for this edition was tape-recorded at the South Miami Child Care Center, where, in the spring of 1980, I spent part of my sabbatical leave from the University of Miami working with four-year-olds in movement. I am primarily indebted to the children with whom I have worked, for their creativity has been the source for most of the ideas found here.

I would like to thank Dr. Joyce McCalla, Director of the Office of Child Development, Dade County Department of Human Resources, Dade County, Florida, for arranging for me to give an in-service training program for child care workers at the South Miami Child Care Center. I would like to acknowledge also the director of the center, Margaret Staples, and the teachers with whom I worked, Theresa Allen, Maria French, Carol Harris, Carolyn Samuel, and Cassandra Smith. Students in a children's literature class taught by Arnold Cheyney at the University of Miami helped with the annotated bibliography of children's books in the Appendix. I would like to thank Ilien Muller-Hechtman,

Barbara Shtupak, and Susan L. Witten for their help, and also Arnold Cheyney for his cooperation.

Photographs from G. Howard Sweet of Miami are used in this edition by permission of the photographer and also from the Permissions Department of Prentice-Hall who own the rights to *The Learning Match* (1980) where these pictures first appeared. Mr. Sweet's ability to catch children in motion cannot be equalled.

I am forever grateful to those who launched my career in higher education: Dr. Alice Miel, the late Dr. Kenneth Wann, and my friend, Edith Weber. *Learning Through Movement* was my first writing in the field of education, and I am glad for this opportunity to revise and update it.

Betty Rowen

Introduction

From the First Edition

*C*hildren love to move. If we watch them at play, we are sure to observe their enjoyment of physical activity. Their faces are animated; their whole bodies are awake and full of life. There is a strong rhythmic quality in their chanting games, their rope skipping, and their ball bouncing. Their play is very much like dancing.

The five-year-old is actually doing a dance step as he skips. Three-year-olds, lacking the coordination to hop on one foot, gallop in the same rhythm instead of skipping. Yet, when they reach nine or ten, children seem to lose some of their agility and freedom. The desire for movement is still there; indeed, large-muscle activity is a major area of interest for them. But too often they have little opportunity to use these large muscles during the school day. All interests thrive on the opportunity to achieve. The nine-year-old has lost not only some of his coordination and joy of movement through disuse, but also a channel of communication with the outside world. For, just as a baby learns through play activity, the school-age child can learn more about reality and his relationship to it through movement.

More opportunity for large-muscle activity is needed for chil-

dren in the elementary grades. They want to move, and movement can be a way to enhance their learning. The teacher in the
primary classroom knows how difficult it is to get her children to sit
still for any length of time. They squirm and they wiggle. Even if
they try hard, they lose interest when they remain inactive for
long. Their faces give back a blank stare, not at all like the
animation we see when they are moving about!

Why can't we let children move? Of course, we cannot have
them running and jumping around the classroom whenever they
like! But we can make constructive use of their innate desire for
movement and let body expression be a part of the learning
process. Ideas that have been discussed in class take on new
meaning when children express them in movement. A story, a
science idea, an incident from history can be dramatized. As
children work with rhythmic patterns in movement, new understandings of number concepts will evolve. When a unit is nearing
completion, a culminating program involving the children in
movement will help to set ideas, and new relationships and insights can be perceived.

If you are a primary school teacher, you may recognize in the
following chapters things you have been doing all along. You may
not have thought you were employing creative movement, or
teaching dance, yet these are some of the same devices used to
develop improvisation in dancers or actors.

The purpose of this book is not to claim movement as a
panacea. Movement is simply another way to reach children, an
avenue that intrigues and invites them. Why not ask your class to
explore one of these avenues with you? Choose any area of the
curriculum you wish. Do you feel that social studies sessions have
been rather dull lately? Are your children understanding all that
they should in language arts? Any area will be livelier when you
introduce interpretive movement into your teaching.

Since movement is a prime motivating force, since it is one
more way for the child to make contact with reality, we cannot
afford to overlook its possibilities in teaching. It has become

standard procedure in classrooms to use materials such as film-strips, tape-recorders, movies, and television as aids to teaching. We do not hesitate to appeal to the child through his eyes and his ears, but we still keep him in his seat. The sense of movement, the kinesthetic sense, is another channel through which we can reach children. We can make good teaching better by employing another area of sensory perception in communicating with children and in developing their powers of communication.

In this book, we will examine movement as being part of an over-all approach to creative teaching. Many illustrations will be given to show movement as part of classroom activity. The discussion of curriculum areas does not mean to imply that this is the only way these subjects are to be presented to children, nor is it necessary to use these methods in every curriculum area. It may be that one of our suggestions will start you thinking of ideas of your own and of ways to implement your own class program through movement. Some idea of how to get started is given in Chapter 1, which describes the process and method of working. Records, books, and stories mentioned in the text are listed at the end of the book. Each teacher, once she is aware of the possibilities, can use movement in her own way.

An Update for the Second Edition

The first edition of this book was written from the perspective of a classroom teacher who had experience as a dancer and dance teacher. This second edition, almost twenty years later, is seen from the point of view of a professor of early childhood education. In the intervening years, I have given numerous workshops for teachers, have demonstrated with children from nursery age through primary grades, have done Head Start training sessions, and have taught prospective teachers of young children on the college campus.

My feeling about the need to expand the use of movement as a means of learning has not changed. To keep children alert and interested in learning, they need the opportunity to move. Learning becomes integrated into an individual as he or she becomes involved in some form of personal expression. "The child's mind is not a passive receptacle into which information can be poured. It is an active, organizing, dynamic system that interacts with its environment throughout the growth process."[1]

The Swiss psychologist, Jean Piaget, has lent support to the premise that activity is essential in learning. Children must act upon their environment. They "assimilate" knowledge only when they can make that information part of themselves by actively becoming involved with it. "Accommodation" takes place as the organism (the child) changes something in its own make-up as a result of stimulation from the environment. That change can take place only through involvement of the self. In the early stages of development, according to Piaget, the child integrates the sensations from the various senses through motor activity. Thus, this first level of development is known as the "sensori-motor" stage.

As a classroom teacher in the early sixties, I did not know about Piaget's work. An astute observer of child behavior, Piaget developed theories concerning how young children learn that lend support to the perceptions of a dance teacher. Learning through movement provides an important method whereby young children may be educated.

Other developments in the area of child study have added to my initial commitment to promote movement as a way of learning. Perceptual-motor training is now considered a factor in the development of prereading skills. Marianne Frostig[2] and others have

---

[1]Betty Rowen, *The Learning Match: A Developmental Guide to Teaching Young Children* (Englewood Cliffs, N.J.: Prentice-Hall, 1980), p. 9.
[2]Marianne Frostig, *The Frostig Program for the Development of Visual Perception* (Chicago: Follett Publishing, 1964).

initiated programs to enhance movement skills in order to help children with learning problems to take the first steps in reading. It is widely recognized that perceptual-motor problems that affect reading and writing may result from deficiencies in body awareness.

In the late sixties, research related to deprivation seemed to point to lack of self-concept as a primary cause for slow learning patterns. Head Start children were found to be uncertain of their own identity. Games in which body parts are named, movements involving body-part isolation, finger plays, and songs with gestures help deprived children to know who they are and what they can do. These findings also support the need for movement experiences in the lives of children. The chapter that follows gives activities to heighten self-concept in young children.

In recent years, added emphasis has been placed upon learning in the first three years of life. Burton White claims that "the period that starts at eight months and ends at three years is a period of primary importance in the development of a human being."[3] Games played at home and at preschool centers affect a child's self-perception. The child develops attitudes toward learning that influence later school experiences.

With this increased interest in the very young child, there is a need for more information about suitable learning activities for this age level. The attention of twos, threes, and fours cannot be maintained for long unless the children are involved in activity. For this reason, I have added to some chapters excerpts from direct dialogues of teachers and young children participating in movement sessions at a child care center.

Throughout, this revision of *Learning Through Movement* reflects the increased awareness that resulted from some of the findings cited above, as well as the additional experiences accumulated as a professional in the field of early childhood education and

[3]Burton White, *The First Three Years of Life* (Englewood Cliffs, N.J.: Prentice-Hall, 1975), p. 4.

child development. My own convictions have been strengthened, and it is hoped that others involved in working with young children will be inspired and motivated to try movement activities as a way of learning.

1 ❧
Beginning Movement Experiences

A basic premise in education is to begin where a child is. The young child is concerned with self and views the world and everything in it in terms of how it relates to him or her. A little girl, for example, can be heard to say, "The sun is following me." The point of reference is the child's own experience, and other objects, such as the sun, are invested with the same responses that the child herself has had.

It is logical, therefore, to begin movement activities with a focus upon the self. We can look at the natural movements of young children and encourage them to expand these movements. Certain basic axial and locomotor movements occur frequently in natural play activity. Children use bouncing movements, often developing into small galloping steps when they are happy or excited. They swing their arms freely as they stand in line waiting for directions from the teacher. Spinning and twisting are fun to do, and ellicit squeals of delight from three-year-olds.

Identifying Body Parts

Natural body movements can be used to begin a movement session. Children can learn to identify body parts as they bounce to a lively beat of a drum or to some strongly rhythmic music.

1

A class of three-year-olds at a child care center was asked to sit around the edge of the rug and listen as the teacher played a record of Nigerian drum music. The children found it hard to sit still as the music built in volume and tempo. The teacher suggested that they imagine that they had a ball to bounce with various parts of their bodies. First they were to use their hands to bounce the ball off the wall. Then they tried to bounce the imaginary ball off the ceiling. Other directions were:

> Bounce it with your elbow.
> Now the other elbow.
> Can you make your head bounce?
> Make your shoulders bounce.
> Make your knees bounce.
> Make your ankles bounce.
> Bounce any part of your body; move around the room.
> Now keep on bouncing and sit down.
> Keep something bouncing until the music stops.

Seated on the floor, the children were asked to point to each part of their bodies as the teacher called them out: head, elbow, knees, ankles (they did not know this one), hands, hips, and so forth.

"Find Another Way to Stretch"

Another activity can begin with stretching exercises to "see how tall you can be." After stretching up high, the children may be directed to fall down to the floor, and to get up slowly and make the stretch get bigger and bigger.

Now, as each child develops his or her stretch, the teacher might ask, "Can you find another way to stretch? How else can you do it?" Different patterns may result. One child may stretch sideways; another may stretch with one arm going up and the other reaching down toward the floor. There is no right or wrong way to do it. The children invent their own stretch movements.

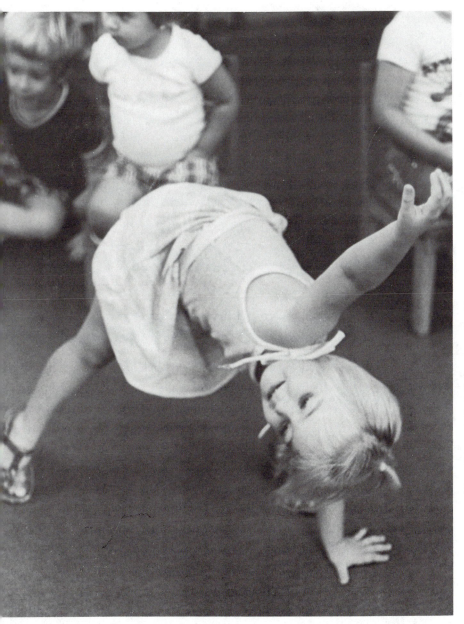

"How many ways can you stretch?"

In a Head Start class in an inner-city school, I used the class of children to demonstrate activities for teachers. The children did not know me, but all responded enthusiastically to the suggestion that they find another way to stretch. Several weeks later, I visited the school again. I was stopped in the hallway by one of the Head Start youngsters. "Look," he said, "I found another way to do it!" And he demonstrated a new stretch he had found. There was excitement and pride in his discovery. The Head Start teacher told me later that this was a child who rarely volunteered to contribute to class discussion. Perhaps the movement idea increased his self-concept, and thus he was able to show what he could do.

Pride in Accomplishment

Pride in physical accomplishment is a characteristic of healthy three- and four-year-olds. The child who gets to the top of the jungle gym for the first time may be heard to exclaim, "Look at me! Look what I can do!" This is a good time to teach tumbling—doing somersaults that go forwards or backwards. Any new physical endeavor builds a feeling of accomplishment.

Four-year-olds begin to be competitive. They can be heard to say, "I can run faster than you!" or "I can climb higher!" Each child can find one or two activities in which to excel, even if it is a small thing like being able to spread fingers apart in the middle! What is important is that youngsters begin to recognize that they have control over their own bodies, and each individual can do what he or she wants with it.

Using Rhythm Instruments

Rhythm instruments provide another way to begin movement. Children are used to "playing in time with the music" in kindergarten, but there are many more things that can be done at various

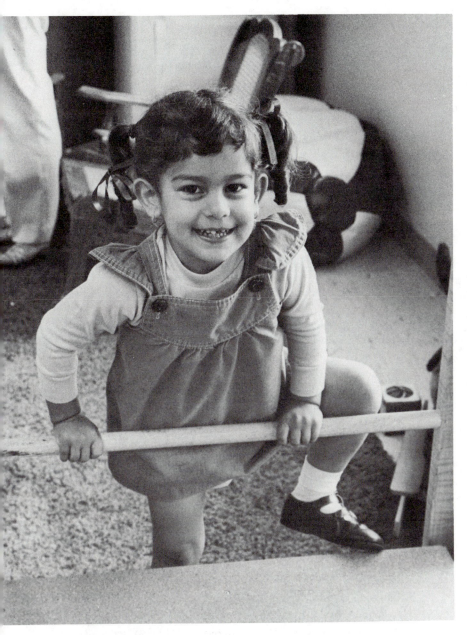

Climbing builds self-concept in three-year-olds. Physical accomplishments lead to joy and a sense of competence, as the child thinks, "Look what I can do!"

grade levels. Children learn to accompany the tempo and rhythm of another child's movement on their drums. They can orchestrate a rhythm, with various instruments playing different parts, while a few children move to the orchestration. In the upper grades, identifying with ethnic groups (Latin American, African, Hindu, for example) adds interest to both the rhythm activity and the social studies program. Even those few who might resist dancing will usually participate eagerly when percussion instruments are made available.

It is a good idea to start a beginner group (any age) by asking them to walk in a circle and to keep time with the teacher's drumbeat. When the beat is fast, the children move quickly around the circle; as it slows down, the children must adjust their tempo as they walk. "The drum is talking to you. You must do as it tells you," a teacher might say to a class of lower graders. "As the drumbeat gets faster, you will go faster. That's right! Now you are running. Listen now. What will the drum do next?"

Children quickly learn to distinguish the uneven beat of a skip or gallop, from the even walk or run. Their feet pick up the pattern established by the drum—ba-DUM, ba-DUM, ba-DUM. . . . They are released and free as they gallop and skip about the room. There is a physical enjoyment of movement that shows on their faces as well as their bodies. The drum slows up. It comes to a stop, and the children stop with it. They all sit on the floor to rest and catch their breath.

Next the teacher might distribute instruments. The children practice keeping time with a leader. They play faster and slower, just as the teacher did before. Then the teacher says to a strongly rhythmic child, "All right, Mark, you may play your own rhythm. Remember to make some accents, some beats that are stronger than others. Try it until you get something you like. Then play it again and again."

A good rhythmic pattern is soon established; the others join in. Most of the group play Mark's rhythm with him. A few may try to improvise one that goes with it. They don't realize what they are

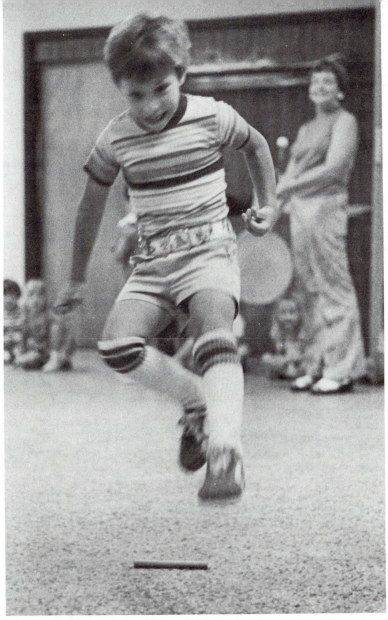

"The drum is talking to you."

doing. They are just "keeping time," but sometimes very interesting combinations are the result. The cymbals may come in only for the accent. The blocks may come in on every other beat. The teacher watches and listens. He or she is quick to spot a rhythmic pattern that blends with the original one, and may suggest orchestrating it, so that one group plays one rhythm while another works in with its own. The children hear the combination and are fascinated. Soon they can direct the orchestration themselves. The child who originates a rhythm usually has a plan for the group to follow.

A good rhythm sets feet tapping, and heads bobbing. "Susan may dance to it," the teacher says. Susan puts down her drum, but the rhythm is still with her. It is all around her as the group continues to play. Soon she is moving, accenting with her body instead of on the drum. With the simple rhythmic pattern to follow, there is unconscious form in her movement. Others join her, each doing their own dances, but all relating to the strong beat of the rhythm band. What a variety of movements are seen! Yet each has a relationship to the rhythm. They are moving differently, but they are together. Sometimes the teacher points out interesting movements but usually saves any comments for later, if all the dancers are absorbed in their dancing.

On some other day, the activity may be worked in reverse. Children create rhythmic patterns as they move. Others accompany them with instruments. The drum helps establish a pattern for the dancer. Sometimes they "follow the leader," who sets the rhythm for the orchestra and the other dancers.

Developing Sensory Awareness

A primary requirement for creativity at any age is that a person be open to new sensations, that he or she perceive with all the senses, and that there be a willingness to take in all observations. In order to "let it all in," the senses need to be sharpened and developed.

In a four-year-old group at a child care center, the children were familiar with following drum beats. The teacher introduced a new percussion instrument, a large Chinese gong. Here is the dialogue that followed:

TEACHER: Listen to my gong.

CHILD: I hear that noise.

TEACHER: Do you want to hear me stop it right away? (Places hand on drum.) What makes it stop?

CHILDREN: Your hand!

TEACHER: Do you want to make it stop? Lie down, and I'll let you feel it. [When children are lying still, they can sense the vibration better.] What does it feel like?

RANDALL: Klingaling.

ADRIENNE: I feel the music!

TEACHER: That's a good way to describe it. Klingaling! The word we use is "vibration." Can you say that?

CHILDREN: Vibration.

TEACHER: That's what makes the sound, and when you put your hand on it, it stops the sound. Now I want you to make a big movement when you hear the gong, and then let it get quieter when the gong gets softer. And stop when the gong stops. It's like melting. Do you know something that melts?

CHILDREN: Ices!

TEACHER: Now let's walk when you hear the gong. And when the gong goes fast and loud, you will go fast. And when the gong goes slow, you go slow. But keep moving slowly until you hear the last sound of the gong.

Through sensory stimulation, the children's creativity is

stimulated. Randall made up a word that described the feeling of the vibration of the gong. He said it felt like "klingaling". The teacher told him that it was called "vibration," but she recognized that "klingaling" possibly described the sensation better!

An alert teacher takes every opportunity to develop sensory awareness by calling attention to sounds and sights, and making children aware of textures, tastes, and smells. Questions like, "How does it make you feel?" "Do you smell anything?" and "Feel how bumpy its skin is!" during class discussions or observations remind the children to use their senses. To see that children make close observations during walks and field trips, to remind them to "react " to things, emotionally as well as intellectually, and to encourage them to make good use of all their senses—these are functions of a good teacher.

There are, however, other devices and techniques that can serve to sharpen sensitivity. Simple guessing games in the classroom are "fun" activities that alert children to sensory perception. Most children are acutely aware of what they see, but they do not always notice sounds, smells, tastes, or qualities observed through touch. Games in which children are asked to guess what the teacher has placed in their hands, or how the teacher has made a certain sound, or what they are smelling increase awareness of the senses and what they can convey.

A step beyond the guessing game is to ask children to react to the "feel" of a sensory perception. Since the right words to describe a feeling are sometimes hard to find, the children might be asked to move "the way it makes you feel." Objects might be chosen by the teacher that possess a definite texture; for example, a "fuzzy" peach, a "smooth" piece of velvet, or "prickly" seedpods. These objects are not shown to the children, but they are asked to touch them and to react to their "feel" in movement. The qualities of the resultant movement studies are often so strongly conveyed that they begin to approach a level of artistic expression.

Young children will be able to "catch a quality" in movement that is initiated in many different ways. Colors have qualities that children are responsive to. Usually blue is "quiet," red is "exciting," and yellow is "happy." The teacher should not comment about the possible qualities but simply ask a child to react to "the bright red of Mary's blouse," for example. "Look at the color, and think how it makes you feel," the teacher says. "Who can show us how it makes you feel?"

"It makes me think of a fire-engine!" a child might answer.

Colored scarves evoke sensory responses and stimulate imagination in young children. After the children at the child care center named the colors, they were asked, "How does yellow make you feel?"

CHILDREN: Happy! Gooo—d!

TEACHER: What's yellow? Do you know anything that is yellow?

CHILDREN: The sun!

TEACHER: What else is yellow? You've got a yellow shirt, right! I am going to give you some scarves. I want you to stand up and take a partner. I am going to give you a scarf and you can play with the scarf—like this (demonstrates waving and moving with scarf). (Gives each couple one scarf.) We are going to throw them up in the air and catch them. You can take turns with your partner. Make them float up in the air and down. Do it slowly because the music is slow music. Now let your partner catch it. And now we are going to do some fast things (plays fast music). Now, children, make a circle. One couple at a time may do a scarf dance in the middle of the circle. (Plays mood music.)

An interesting thing happened at the end of this movement session. When the teacher asked the children to take hands in a circle, they began to sing spontaneously:

Good morning to you,
Kenya, Kenya, Kenya.
Good morning to you.
Kenya, how are you?

This is a song that they had learned previously. The children sang to each member of the group, without any direction from the teacher. There was a joyful, friendly feeling as the children addressed each one individually. I strongly believe that the freedom to express feelings started in the movement session and carried over into the spontaneous singing after the class.

Group Improvisations

Sometimes the teacher may get everyone involved by telling a story that has continuity but where the characters create their own parts. Getting children to "feel the part" will be easier as they become freer through movement experiences.

The teacher must set the scene, but what happens after that is left to the individuals who are part of it. The story should present a challenging situation, but the solution should be undefined. Here are two favorite stories that I have worked out with young children and that lend themselves either to dramatization with dialogue or simply to movement with possible background music:

1. *"A Day in the Park."*   Children come to the park to play. They come through a gate, one at a time. (The teacher can be the gatekeeper, or even the rotating turnstile!) They play in various ways in the playground. Some ride on swings, some on see-saws. As they play, other people enter—a lady with a baby carriage, an old man, and so forth. A policeman helps a lost boy to find his mother. A girl expects to meet a friend who doesn't come. Various situations can be invented by the children. A rainstorm sends them all rushing for cover. (The music "Golliwoggs's Cakewalk"

seems to make a natural accompaniment for this action[1].)

2. *"The Scarecrow."* A boy wants to go to a fair, but his mother will not allow him to go. (Mother may invent her own reason.) He decides to run away, but he gets lost in the woods on the way. He sits down to rest, falls asleep, and a witch who knows that he is being bad casts a spell on him. When he awakens, he is stiff and unable to move. He is a scarecrow. Various people then pass through the woods on their way to the fair. They are surprised to see a scarecrow in the woods, and each reacts differently. Children may invent their own characters, possibly a clown who works at the fair, a playful boy, a lonesome girl, the boy's mother. The end of the story can be created by the players as well.

The teacher need not hesitate to make suggestions as the story progresses. Although taking part in the fun of the activity, the teacher should remain alert to direct and supervise when necessary. And it is the teacher who decides what is the best place to stop.

Sometimes a story written by a child lends itself well to dramatization. A boy in the third grade wrote:

> I wanted to go with my father to work one day. He would not take me. After he left, I got on the train after him. I didn't want him to see me. Then I lost him. I didn't know where to get off. Who will help me?

We tried acting out this story and found that it was very good for dramatization. Various children became the different people on the train: the conductor, a nice old lady, a grouchy man. Our solution came when the boy found one of his mother's friends on the train, and she stopped at the next station to call his mother on the telephone. Perhaps another class would find a different ending.

---

[1]"Golliwogg's Cakewalk" is a selection in Debussy's *Children's Corner Suite* (see Appendix C).

Upper graders in the elementary school may take a little longer to develop spontaneity in movement. Rhythm instruments may seem like "baby stuff" to them, and dancing is "taboo" for boys of this age. But fourth and fifth graders love to dramatize scenes from history. They also enjoy strong work movements and rhythmic activity that is related to sports they know.

The train story mentioned above can be adapted to use with older children as well. Various characters and situations on the train can be enacted. A crowded city street, a scene in a Paris cafe (or located in whatever country the class has been studying) all lend themselves to the introduction of various distinct characters. The teacher need not invent the characters but should very carefully set the scene, so that a real place is envisioned.

Children of this age love mystery and suspense, so a favorite theme is finding a mysterious box in the attic or getting a secret package. Here again, either pure movement with musical background or improvisation with dialogue can be successful. It may be better to have movement without speech until the group has developed enough concentration to work well.

Fifth graders may enjoy "playing" a baseball game, where only the bat and ball are missing! The action of each player is made clear through pantomime. The children relate to each other, throwing and catching an imaginary ball. The teacher may pick up the underlying beat of their movements on a drum. He or she encourages them to exaggerate the important movements, leave out those that do not heighten the essential qualities of the "baseball game." The results can be a group dance of real quality. This baseball game is played, not to teach baseball (although it could do just that), but as a way of freeing older children for movement. They enjoy this activity. They discover what fun it is to do rhythmic pantomime.

Creative movement may evolve into dances, but it is closely related to drama as well. The teacher may begin with a pantomime of everyday activity. He or she tries to get the children to concentrate on what they are doing, to see imaginary objects as if they really were there, to forget themselves and become absorbed with the person they have become. The teacher can say that "we are acting out" an idea or a story or that "we are moving as if we were" something or someone. It is better to avoid the word "dance" which may create self-consciousness. A good way to start might be to say "Let's see what you have done."

How Creative Movement Evolves in the Classroom

Now let's visit a class that has already been introduced to some creative movement. This is a second grade classroom. Let's see how the movement studies develop during one session. It is mid-morning, and the children who have been working at their seats or at the reading table are beginning to squirm restlessly. It is time for a break.

The chairs and desks are pushed back, clearing as much floor space as possible. The teacher has a drum in one hand, a soft-ended tympany stick in the other. A phonograph stands ready for use, too. The children are permitted to remove their shoes, if they care to. (They usually do.) We are ready to begin.

"Let us stretch way up to the ceiling. Take a deep breath in. Pull up in the middle. Now stretch, get bigger through your whole body. Make your necks long. Now let it all out and drop down!" The teacher's voice and drumbeats build up the feeling. "Now let's grow bigger again starting from the bottom and building up to the head. Stretch . . . and drop!"

So far the teacher has directed the activity. It is not very different from the exercises that are usually given to allow children to stretch between lessons. Actually if you have difficulty following these directions, any stretch exercise would serve to release body tensions, awaken kinesthetic feeling, and bring muscles to life. I know it is not easy to interpret movement patterns from written words, but I hope to convey a way of working. The movements you use can be ones that you are familiar with or that the children do in their gymnasium period.

Next the second-graders do swinging movements that are free and relaxed. They all start together, being led by the strong, rhythmic beat of the drum. But soon the teacher says, "Now swing any way you like! Remember to let it drop down just like the swings in the playground. Try letting your leg be a swing. Now your whole body!" The teacher praises the free movements, and points out new variations.

The drumbeat leads them toward a crescendo and then subsides. The teacher resumes direction again, as the class does little bouncy jumps, pushing off the floor with their toes. "Pull up in the middle. The center of your body is a ball that is bouncing." The directions stress the feeling of the movement.

All members of the class are now participating, for these are enjoyable movements. The children soon forget themselves in the relaxed rhythmic use of their bodies.

They drop to the floor to catch their breath. "What shall we act out today?" the teacher asks. Almost always there is an answer. Sometimes the teacher provokes the thinking. "Did you like the story we read yesterday about the farm? What did the farmer do? No, don't tell us! Let's see if you can show us!" Several children are selected to improvise movements. Some move self-consciously, and their movements are small and tentative. "Make your movements bigger. Think about what you are doing, and let us know what it is."

The others who are watching are allowed to pick out the movements they like and to guess what they are. John is digging toward the ground and swinging his arms up to the side.

"John is pitching hay!" says Mary.

"Good, can you keep time for him on my drum, Mary?" the teacher says. "Make your movements bigger, John. Get your whole body into it."

Several children join John doing his movement. Then the teacher asks, "What other movement did you like?"

"I liked what Alice did when she was on her knees smoothing the ground."

"I wasn't smoothing the ground," says Alice, "I was planting seeds."

"Yes, and we could see that she cared for her work by her gentle movement," says the teacher. "Let's have a few of you on your knees in that corner, planting. John, you and the others with you keep your movement going. Let's see how they look together."

There are other movements. Steven is driving a tractor. He shuffles around, jogging over bumps, rising to his toes and then continuing with knees bent. His rhythm is twice as fast as John's, although both are relating to the drumbeat. The teacher points this out. "Every time John does his movement, Steven takes two steps. See? He is going twice as fast!"

Later, they might count their steps, and the dance might take form. But for now, the teacher wants them to express themselves freely in movement. Counting might spoil this.

"All right, everybody up now. Let's all do some farm work. Yes, you may try John's movement if you like. Good, Susan, that's a new one.

"Now the farmers have finished. They take their tools back to the shed. They are tired, but they feel good because they have worked hard and well. They walk slowly, but with a sure step. They breathe the soft evening air. They smell the hay. They walk back to their house."

The children walk quietly to their seats. In this last moment, they have all been caught up in the mood. Each one is a "farmer" until the last drumbeat is sounded.

After the children have been exposed to movement experiences of this nature, they will be willing to participate in story dramatization and in movement improvisations related to all areas of the curriculum. The chapters that follow give suggestions and examples of learning experiences made more meaningful through movement exploration.

2 ❧
Language and Movement

*M*ovement is important to children, and so it should be important to their teachers as well. A sound approach to any phase of the school curriculum takes into account the child who is to be taught. Because children like to move, and because using their bodies is a natural means of expression for them, a teacher can get a lively response from a class by incorporating movement whether the subject is arithmetic, social studies, or language arts.

For young children, language and movement go together. They move their arms excitedly when they have something to tell us. They are likely to jump up and down when they are happy. Fear and anger show in their whole bodies, and movement accompanies vocalization whenever their emotions are aroused.

The primitive combination of movement and language that young children exhibit can help to heighten sensitivity to the sounds of language. Heightened sensitivity leads naturally to appreciation of the spoken and written word and to response to poetry.

Later I will discuss how movement can implement word study, story comprehension, and other aspects of the language arts program, but we will begin where little children begin, that is, with the sounds of language.

The Sounds of Language

I have asked children in a classroom to do things that might seem a little wild to adults but that seem perfectly natural to the children. I ask them to move around the room in any way they like and to make noises as they go! This is a welcome release, but if we watch closely and listen, we will see an interesting phenomenon. The sounds the children make are perfect accompaniment for their movement. They not only accent the rhythm of what they are doing, but they catch the quality of the movement as well.

Paula is doing a swinging movement, and her hum rises and falls with her arms and body. Perry hisses as he spins around. The hiss grows in intensity as he takes bigger and faster turns. Heidi springs up from all fours and squeaks in a syncopated pattern with her movement. The whole effect is pert and implike.

Other children are doing animal movements. The sounds go with the movement, as when you come to think of it, they do in the animal world as well! The chirp of a bird usually accompanies its hop. The lion roars as it springs. The children in my classroom have the same primitive combination of sound and movement as do the animals they are imitating.

They take turns showing their movements one at a time to the class. There is no self-consciousness. This is natural, everyday activity for the youngsters, and they are quite willing to share this experience with an adult they sense is "going along with them," that is, enjoying their movement exploration in the spirit of fun.

Children have strong intuitive feelings about sounds that go with movements. Watch and listen to children on the playground. A girl hums and sings as she swings back and forth on the swing. Notice the boy who is an airplane. As he banks his arms for the turn, hear his motor soar!

Children in the primary grades are not so far removed from the stage in which sound and movement are one. Their play activity

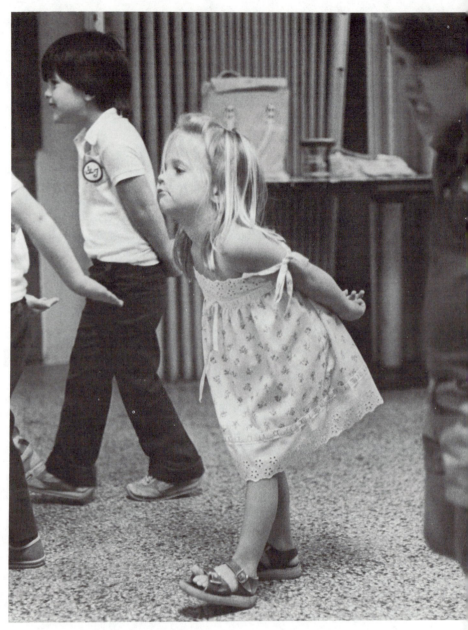

Children imitate animal movements making appropriate sounds to accompany themselves.

makes meaningful use of sounds to accompany movement. We can make the sounds of our language more meaningful to them through movement. This is one device for developing sensitivity to the sound of expressive language.

Vocal sounds have emotional quality. Children can move in a way that expresses how the sound makes them feel. "Ah" often suggests wonder and awe. Usually there is an "opening out" of the arms, a straightening of the back, and a suspended breath quality in the child's movement when moving to the "ahh" sound. We have found that "ee" evokes strong, assertive movements, and "ooh" results in enclosing, circling type of movements. Of course, there are variations, and the feeling conveyed is often a reflection of the teacher's tone of voice in saying the sounds. Nevertheless, there seems to be some consistency in the children's reactions to different sounds. Sounds have qualities, and these qualities can be experienced through movement. A sensitivity to sounds of language is present in children, and can be cultivated. The beauty of language in poetry and prose is dependent largely upon its combination of sounds. Sensitivity to sounds deepens children's potential emotional response to the language arts.

Exploring Natural Body Movement

Movement exploration should begin with natural body movements. These are the things that all children enjoy doing: swinging, stretching, jumping, galloping. An imaginary trip to a park or playground gives children a chance to explore natural body movements in time to the teacher's drum or piano. Such an imaginary trip was taken by a group of four-year-olds at a day care center in a poverty area. A transcript of their movement session follows:

TEACHER: Let's stand up and stretch. Let's see how big you can be. Let's stretch all the way up to the sky. When you stretch, can you make your neck long? Pull your shoulders down and stretch way up. Take a deep breath. In—and fall down (strong beat on drum). Now let's get bigger and bigger—and stretch. And fall down! And get bigger again. Stretch all the way up to the sky. And this time you're not going to fall all the way to the ground. You're going to drop down and come right up again like a swing. Ready? Down and up! Down and up!

CHILDREN: Down and up! Down and up!

TEACHER: (Plays swing rhythm on drums.) Good! Watch Ricki; that's very good. When you are on a swing, it doesn't stop at the bottom, does it? It drops down and comes right up again, right? Let's see you try it. Make it go down and right back up again. (Plays swinging rhythm.) When you are on the playground, can you swing by yourself or does someone have to push you?

CHILD: I can swing all by myself!

TEACHER: Good. And when you bend your knees, that makes your swing go higher, doesn't it? Swing and bend your knees. Look at Zira. That's beautiful! Now try to walk around as you swing. Go. Let your arms swing. Now turn around and face the middle of the circle. We're going to swing into the circle and back from the circle. Swing up and down! That's beautiful. Now swing your arms anyway you want to swing them, but keep them going! Watch Kenya swing. She has a different way to swing them. Watch Shiriba swing. Beautiful. Find another way. She's swinging her arms around, like she's swinging a lasso. Yes, you can turn around, too. I'm going to say a poem about a swing, and then we're going to swing to it:

How do you like to go up in a swing?
Up in the air so blue?
Oh, I do think it the pleasantest thing
Ever a child can do![1]

Put one foot in front of the other, and step forward
and back as you swing. Go. (Repeats poem.) Now
let's hop up in the air as we step forward onto the
front foot:

Up in the air and over the wall,
Till I can see so wide,
Rivers and trees and cattle and all
Over the countryside—

Can you look down and do a low swing? This is like
Kenya's swing. It's a low swing that goes around
your body (demonstrates).

Till I look down on the garden green
Down on the roof so brown—
Up in the air I go flying again,
Up in the air and down!

Wasn't that a nice poem?
All right. Now let's take a partner. Put your two
hands together like this. (Makes pairs, partners
facing each other.) Do you know what we are going
to do? We're going to make a see-saw—like in the
playground. As one side goes up, the other side
goes down (demonstrates with a child). Did you

[1]Robert Louis Stevenson, "The Swing," *A Child's Garden of Verses* (New
York: Random House, 1978), p. 11.

ever go on a see-saw in the park? When one side
goes down, what does the other side do?

CHILDREN: Goes up! Goes down!

TEACHER: Let's do it together. When one side goes up the other
side goes down. Change! Let's say, seesaw,
seesaw. (Children chant.) Change, change. One
side goes up, the other goes down.

All of the things we were doing today are things that
you do when you go to the playground in the park.
What other things are there to do at the park?

CHILD: Sliding board!

TEACHER: Let's climb up the steps—and slide down! Good.

Now let's all walk to the park. And we're so happy
we're going to skip! And now we're at the park.
Let's all get on a swing. And go down and up! What
would you like to go on next? A see-saw. All right,
get your partner. One side goes up and one side
goes down. Watch Ricki and Celia! Very good.
Now everybody do it.

Did you have a good time at the playground?

CHILDREN: Yes!

TEACHER: Let me ask you something. Did we really go to the
playground today?

CHILDREN: [Some answer yes; some no.]

TEACHER: Were we really at the playground, or were we making
believe?

CHILD: Making believe!

TEACHER: Yes, we were making believe. But it was almost like
real because we did all the things we would do if we
really went there. You really made believe very
well.

Dramatizing Past Experiences

Another imaginary trip might be taken to the circus. If some of the children have already been to the circus, they love to tell what they saw there. Plans for movement sessions should relate to children's real experiences. If the circus is in town, then that is the time for movement exploration about circus themes.

In one class the teacher began by asking what the children saw at the circus. They answered:

"Clowns—they did funny tricks."
"A man went flying through the air."
"Elephants—he put a man up in the air."
"Horses, with people standing on them."

There was much excitement in relaying this information, and it was difficult to get children to talk one at a time. The teacher reviewed the signal for stopping (putting a drum stick in air) and asked children to stop talking and "freeze" at signal.

The class got up to walk in a circle and "listen for drum-talk." Children did walks, runs, tiptoe steps, and giant steps. They were then introduced to uneven drum beats. They did not know what the drum was telling them to do, so the teacher suggested galloping like horses in the circus. When the drum stopped, they were to stand still and try to balance on one foot, like a bareback rider. The children did the activity several times. Then they were asked to walk like elephants, taking "big heavy steps." Some made their arms swing like the trunks of an elephant. The teacher said, "Make your trunk swing," but did not specify how they should do this.

Everyone then had a chance to be a "funny clown." Children made a circle, and three children were asked to go into the middle and do funny tricks. Then three more children were chosen. Many made funny faces and jumped around. The teacher asked if any of the clowns did handstands or cartwheels. After that, all of the "clowns" did acrobatic tricks. Many were able to do good cartwheels and could stand on their hands briefly.

The children practiced making a "swing" as they had done at a previous session. The teacher then suggested that they pretend they were on a "flying trapeze" like the performers in the circus. They were to swing three times and then fly through the air. Children were lined up in two lines, and as they flew through the air, they were to change places. They had difficulty avoiding bumping into each other as they flew through the air!

They were then asked to sit down on the rug to rest and to talk about what they did.

Experiences such as these lead to language development. The children are eager to share the excitement of their circus visit. Social skills are learned as they take turns telling about what they saw. An experience chart may be made, using the children's own verbal language. Even though the children may not be able to read what has been written, they learn to identify the written symbols with ideas they have expressed.

Word Study

Teachers spend much time in the primary grades helping children develop a "sight vocabulary." Children learn to recognize whole words as they appear in sentences. Experience charts can be used to build sentences about experiences in the classroom or on a trip. That is fine, but there are other ways to clarify word meanings. Do the first-graders who read, "Look, Sally, see Spot run" know the distinction between "look" and "see," for instance? Acting out these words is another way to make meaningful associations for the beginning reader.

Later, we teach the endings that are added to words: -ing, -ed, -ly, and so forth. The children may know that they must drop the "silent e" when adding "ing," but do they know the difference between "hiding" and "hidden"?

To illustrate, in a second-grade class I was helping the children act out words from a new vocabulary list for a reading lesson one

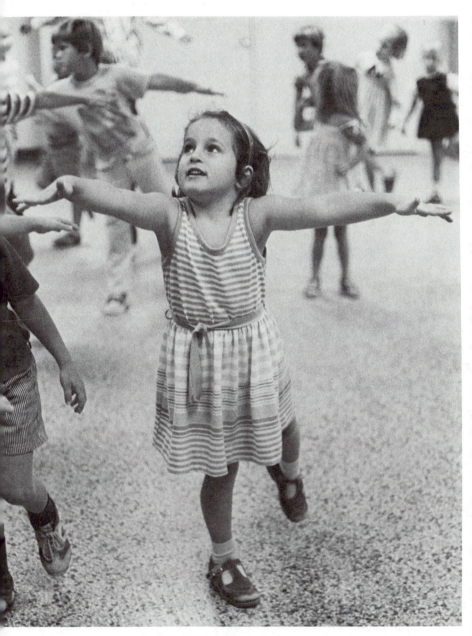

Balancing on one foot is an essential perceptual-motor skill, but moving the way a bare-back rider in the circus does make this exercise more fun!

day. For the word "sleepy," Sandy lay on the floor with eyes closed, pretending to be asleep.

"Is 'sleepy' the same as 'sleeping'?" I asked. Many children did not know. They talked about it for a while, and then a few of the group offered to act out "sleepy" again. One was an early morning riser, struggling to arise from bed. He tossed and turned on the floor, stretching and yawning, and finally succumbing to the feeling and going back to sleep. Another was doing homework, as the feeling of "sleepy" crept over her. The whole class tried it. They knew what it was to be "sleepy" because they actually were experiencing it in these brief movement studies.

Movement can be a way in which words become a part of the child. Adults so often perceive things from only their own vantage point. They assume that when a child uses a word correctly in a sentence, he or she understands it. We forget the limitations of children's experience. We can broaden that experience through movement. The children described above will always know the difference between "sleepy" and "sleeping" because they felt it with their whole bodies.

Introducing movement had some additional benefits. The children were actively participating in the lesson. Although they were acting "sleepy," their mental processes were very much awake! They were bringing something of themselves, their own interpretation, to the lesson. They were interested because physical involvement always arouses the interest of children. Imaginations were stimulated, too.

For the word, "cold," Ian took an imaginary ice cube from a tray. It slipped from his fingers and went scurrying across the floor. He tried to retrieve it several times, and finally missed his footing and landed on the floor himself!

Everyone laughed. This was a very amusing bit of pantomime, and it was very convincingly done. Ian's concentration was good. He actually felt the coldness of the ice as he handled it, and so did the audience.

"What else did Ian show us about the ice?" I asked. "It was

slippery!" several answered. The meaning of another word was clarified.

Meanings are intensified when words that "describe things" are enacted. Here are some others that have worked well:

bumpy	hot	angry	silly
sticky	damp	happy	lazy
smooth	funny	sad	suddenly

The meaning of the word "suddenly" was not at all clear to one reading group, until Laurie associated it with a story. "Here, I'll show you" she said, and proceeded to act out the "Sing a Song o' Sixpence" rhyme. The group quickly guessed what she was enacting, but they didn't relate it to the new word in the story for the day.

"Don't you see?" Laurie said. "The king opened the pie, and SUDDENLY out flew the birds!"

Action or "doing" words make good dramatization, too. These have been tried successfully:

hiding	skate	squirm	rake
finding	slide	shiver	dig
running	carry	bounce	drop
wiggling	push	jump	sniff
crawling	pull	fly	touch

The distinction can be made between present and past tense, and if the class is ready, spelling changes can be emphasized along with change in meaning. One class knew quite well how to read the words "scare" or "scared." ("A goblin will scare you." "I am scared.") But it wasn't until they acted these two words out, that they sensed what a big difference there was in their meanings!

Let's not forget that children can "be" as well as "do" different things. Nouns can be used for action as well. For example:

bird	cat	ocean
airplane	elephant	leaves
boat (different kinds)	mouse	snowflakes
fire	wind	steam shovel

Generally whatever words are new in a reading or in a class discussion may be enacted. The teacher may point to a new word on the blackboard and ask one or all the children to act it out. Or a "charade" game may be played. A list of new words is put on the board. A child chooses one, shows it to the class in movement, and the rest must guess. The first child who guesses the correct word may then act out another word. The teacher should emphasize that the purpose of this game is to "do the word so well that we can all guess quickly," and set a time limit during which the word must be guessed or the performer must sit down.

This game can be used for all kinds of word drill. Suppose the class has learned a new phonics rule, such as "when two vowels walk together, the first one says its name." The list on the board would include:

boat	mail	reach	peal
goat	train	clean	meat
wheel	feed	fear	eat

If this is a spelling lesson, a child who answers might have to spell the word without looking at the list, before getting a chance to act out another word. Almost any group of words in a spelling, phonics, or reading lesson has among them many that lend themselves to action. Meanings will be clarified and intensified, interest will be maintained, and imagination and thought will be stimulated, if the time spent on drill and review involves the children in movement.

At a more advanced level, having students "act out" words can be used to teach parts of speech. The distinction between words that describe things (adverbs and adjectives), "doing words" (verbs), and words that are names of things (nouns) can be made. Moving to these words can make their functions clear.

Appreciating Poetry

Sensitivity to the sounds of language and to the shades of meaning of words heighten children's aesthetic response to literature. If movement can bring new meaning to these elements of language, surely it will be even more effective in making poems and stories "come alive."

The strong rhythmic pattern of some poems for children makes it difficult for them to sit still when someone is reading to them. And why should they? Galloping around the room to "Ride a Cock Horse to Banbury Cross" makes the poem more fun! The teacher can bring out the fact that the rhythmic pattern sounds like a horse galloping. The children may clap the rhythm as others move to it. This is fun, but it is also developing awareness of the rhythmic pattern that is so much part of the beauty of poetry.

All the Mother Goose rhymes are strongly rhythmic, and possibly that is one of the reasons they have been such favorites of children for generations. Action is suggested by many of them, and so when children move as we read to them, they unconsciously set the action to the rhythmic pattern. They are not just "acting out," they are dancing! "Little Miss Muffet" has a truly dynamic quality when children move to it. Of course, two children are needed. As Miss Muffet carefully spoons her "curds and whey" into her mouth, the spider stealthily creeps up on her. The speeded rhythm on "And frightened Miss Muffet away" provides a climax for the movement of the spider (who usually pounces!) and Miss Muffet (who runs away), and a feeling of excitement is communicated to the viewers. "Jack and Jill," "Jack-Be-Nimble," and "Tom, Tom, the Piper's Son" are also favorites for action.

Nursery rhymes are not just for preschool or kindergarten

classes. Sixth-graders have been known to enjoy movement studies based upon them. Older children like to be involved in entertaining the younger ones. An excellent opportunity for bilingual education might occur if sixth-graders acted out nursery rhymes or familiar fairy tales while the accompanying narration is done in Spanish and English.

To encourage respect for cultural differences, songs and chants from other parts of the world, such as Africa, may also be used for movement studies. Vachel Lindsay's "The Congo"[2] makes exciting dramatization for upper grade youngsters. The dynamics of the rhythmic pattern is felt clearly when children move as the teacher reads.

"My Shadow" presents an interesting situation in which children can work in pairs, one as the child and the other as the shadow. Learning to relate to each other in movement is a valuable social and aesthetic experience. The strong beat of the poem keeps the children together or allows them to do a "follow the leader" pattern:

Child A	*Child B*
I have a little shadow	that goes in and out with me,
And what can be the use of him	is more than I can see.
He is very, very like me	from the heels up to the head;
And I see him jump before me,	when I jump into my bed.[3]

On the last line, it might be suggested that Child B (the shadow) take the jumping movement first, with Child A following on the second half of the line. The teacher should refrain from giving too much suggestion of movement, however. Set gestures to this kind of poem could destroy the quality and stifle the children's spont-

---

[2]May be found in Louis Untermeyer, ed., *Modern American Poetry* (New York: Harcourt, Brace & World, 1962).
[3]Stevenson, "My Shadow," *Child's Garden of Verses*, p. 17.

aneous responses. Those of us who have been doing movement activities with children know that their ideas are much better than ours, anyhow!

A poem often suggests the movement to the children, but in spite of this, no two groups will respond in exactly the same way. Such a poem is Dorothy Aldis' "The Elephants":

> With their trunks the elephants
> Hold hands in a long row—
> Their little eyes so quick and wise
> Their feet so big and slow
> They climb on top of things and then
> When they are told, climb down again.[4]

Stereotyped movements are not easily forgotten, once children have learned them. When they hear "elephant," many youngsters will immediately clasp both hands making a "trunk" and begin swinging arms with heavy steps. We have all seen this conventional interpretation of the elephant walk, and it has long lost its meaning to the child doing it. The teacher might remind the group of the words in the poem. "They hold hands in a long row. Did you ever see how elephants do this?" "Yes, their steps are still 'big and slow' and their trunks swing as they walk, don't they?" Asking the children to recall how elephants move, and then to "show us in your own way," breaks the set response previously learned, and gives truer content to the interpretation of the poem.

Sometimes it is not the rhythm nor the story of a poem that motivates the children to move. It is a quality they are trying to capture. Carl Sandburg's poem "Fog"[5] affects even young first graders. The poem might be read first, and the fog creeping "on little cat feet" might be dramatized to the accompaniment of a tone on the gong or a low quiet rumble on the piano. On a day when

---

[4]Dorothy Aldis, "The Elephants," *All Together* (New York: G. P. Putnam's Sons, 1952), p. 129.

[5]May be found in Untermeyer, ed., *Modern American Poetry*.

children have come to school through a fog, what better way is there for them to sense the picture image of the poem? Some lead-up discussion as to "what the fog made you think of," and so on, is good. Perhaps the dramatization with the musical sounds should precede reading the poem. This is something for a teacher to decide.

Children have favorite characters in poems and stories, and they love to pretend that they are Christopher Robin or Winnie-the-Pooh. The poems of A. A. Milne might accompany their actions or might simply serve as inspiration for their own story ideas involving the characters.

These are classroom activities whose sole purpose is to heighten the meaning of poetry for children. The resultant movement studies need not have value as performance pieces. An attempt to orient the child toward preparing for an audience sometimes destroys the qualities we are trying to develop. They do, however, show their studies to others in the class, and the reaction of their classmates is a good indication of the effectiveness of the piece as communication. If "something good" is produced in this way, it might be nice to show it to others at an assembly program or to invite another class to view it.

Sometimes a poem can be developed into a production involving the entire school. Robert Browning's poem *The Pied Piper of Hamelin* was a favorite of a sixth-grade class. They liked to read it and talk about the characters, since they had a student council of their own. "Imagine those snooty councilmen deciding not to pay the poor Piper," one child commented. "I can just see them shooing him away, and acting so proud of themselves!" "Show me," the teacher said, and that was how it all started.

Soon swaggering councilmen were parading all over the room. The teacher reached for her drum to set a rhythm for them. "I like the way Neal carries his head. That hand movement is good, Tom." It was amazing how many characterizations there were, and some were very funny. Some children seem to have a natural feeling for satirical pantomime.

The class improvised movement for all the characters of the story. Each day they tried a different part. They talked about how the Piper looked and how he moved as he played his pipe. They talked about how the rats scurried about. They tried being the rats. They talked about the children playing together and about how they were fascinated by the Piper and led away. They acted out the scene. They talked about the way the people felt when their children left them. They did sad, grieving movements.

The group decided to do this last scene, standing together, using a swaying motion. Then one "mother" came forward and did a movement of her own to express her grief, while the group swayed behind her. She returned and another came forward, doing a different movement. The pattern for the dance was established, although the individual movements were different each time they were done. It didn't matter. The children knew the story and remembered the people they were portraying. They gave convincing performances each time.

The class asked if the dramatization could be shown to the entire school. They decided that before each scene a narrator should read the part of the poem that explained the action. The music teacher cooperated, and discovered some piano selections from Bela Bartok's "Children's Pieces" that made excellent accompaniment for the movement.

All the children tried all the parts. After a while they agreed that some were better as councilmen and others were convincing as the grieving parents.

"Wouldn't it be nice if we could get some of the lower-graders to be the children?" one grown-up sixth-grader suggested.

"They would be good as the rats, too," said another.

A committee was sent to the kindergarten teacher to explain the situation. She was glad to cooperate, and she told the kindergarten children the story.

What wonderful rats they made! They scurried about with quick, darting motions, and seemed much more at ease on all fours than the bigger children had been.

They were good in the children's scene, too. They did some of the things they had done before in their kindergarten rhythms sessions. They made "swings" and played "sail-a-boat," they skipped and ran. When the Piper came, they really seemed to be charmed by him. They didn't have to remember their dances because the Pied Piper, a sixth-grader, was there to lead them.

Other classes heard of the sixth-grade project. The third-graders had learned a Bavarian folk dance. They wondered if they could do it in one of the scenes. It fit very well into the scene where the townspeople were celebrating the removal of the rats. The third-graders were part of the celebration.

When the performance in the auditorium finally came, there were as many involved in the show as there were in the audience. It is better that way. Involvement means remembering, and none of these children will ever forget Browning's classic narrative poem.

Story Dramatization

Acting out stories helps children remember the sequence of events and understand characters and meanings. This seems to be particularly true when fairy tales are acted out in preschool.

A research study by Eli Saltz of Wayne State University, provides evidence that children who act out fairy tales in preschool on a regular basis do better in elementary school than youngsters who haven't had such experience. According to Saltz, these children consistently scored ten points higher on intelligence tests, and at ages eight and nine they excelled at tasks requiring a grasp of concepts. Saltz's study results were repeated three times in separate experiments, and his four-year follow-up confirmed the widespread and continuing influence of fairy-tale theater activity in preschool.[6]

[6]"Researcher Claims Preschoolers' 'Acting Experience' Affects Elementary School Work," *Today's Child News Magazine* 28, no. 5 (May 1980).

I was able to substantiate Saltz's evidence in working with preschoolers in a day care center in a poverty area. The children were given an opportunity to act out parts of the story of "Jack and the Beanstalk." They dramatized the sequence of events with all the children enthusiastically playing the various roles:

Jack pulled the cow on a rope and took him to the market.
A man [the teacher] gave Jack colored beans for the cow.
Jack planted the colored beans.
Children became the beans growing out of the ground.
Jack climbed the beanstalk.
Everyone tiptoed as if walking on a cloud.
They knocked on the door of the castle.
The giant came out, took giant steps, and said,
    "Fe fi fo fum, I am a giant, and here I come!"
Jack ran away.
They repeated giant steps and Jack's running steps.
Jack climbed down the beanstalk.
Jack got a hatchet and chopped down the beanstalk.
The giant fell into a hole.

At a movement session several weeks later, the children were asked to recall what they had done. A transcript of their conversation follows:

TEACHER: How much do you remember about the story of "Jack and the Beanstalk?" What did we do first?

CHILDREN: We made a bean . . . . We made a bean pole. We put some beans in the ground. You gave us a cow.

TEACHER: And I gave you some beans for the cow and you went home and . . .

CHILD: Planted them in our garden.

TEACHER: Yes, and what happened next?

CHILDREN: They growed and growed—and growed.

TEACHER: All the way up to the . . .

CHILDREN: Sky!

TEACHER: And then you were Jack, and what did Jack do?

CHILD: He climbed up the beanstalk.

TEACHER: And then what happened?

CHILD: We knocked very hard on the door.

TEACHER: But before you knocked on the door, what did we walk on?

CHILDREN: Clouds!

TEACHER: We walked on the clouds, and we had to walk carefully and very softly on clouds. Then we got to the door and who came out?

CHILDREN: Giant!

TEACHER: And he said, "Fie fie foe fum, I am a giant, and here I come!"
[Children joined in.] What did Jack do?

CHILDREN: Run!

TEACHER: Ran away and the giant ran after him. Then Jack climbed down the beanstalk. And then what happened?

CHILDREN: We chopped, chopped, chopped.

TEACHER: What happened to the giant?

CHILDREN: He died.

TEACHER: He fell into the hole and he died. You remember everything so well!

The children in this class had the limited language ability

usually associated with deprivation of experience. Yet they were able to express themselves well and could tell the story in the sequence in which they had acted it out several weeks before. Very often children, when asked to tell about a story that had been read to them, will tell the part most important to them first. They might say, "The giant got killed!" But these children were able to answer my questions and could tell what happened first, second, and "after that" with no difficulty.

Story dramatization can also help children develop understanding of descriptive words that are not usually part of their vocabulary. A story that I have used frequently for this purpose is about a toy rocking horse. Some children have never seen one, and so it is important to demonstrate how the horse rocks on its rockers, perhaps using a rocking chair to illustrate. Then the children do the rocking movement.

TEACHER: How can you rock? I don't want you to rock in the chair. I want you to rock by yourself. Good! That's a good way to rock? Look how Kayla is rocking? Do you all have to rock the same way? Look at Aaron. He's on his knees and rocking. Let's try Aaron's way to rock. Look at Kimberly. Roll all the way back and put your feet over your head like Kimberly did. Lie on your stomachs now and hold onto your feet. I'm going to give you a ride. Now can you do it by yourself?

Here is a song about a rocking horse:

> I'm rocking rocking all the time;
> I wish that I could move.
> I'm rocking rocking all the time
> In the same old grove.
> I wish that I could go someplace;
> I'd like to run away.
> But here I always have to stay
> And rock and rock all day.

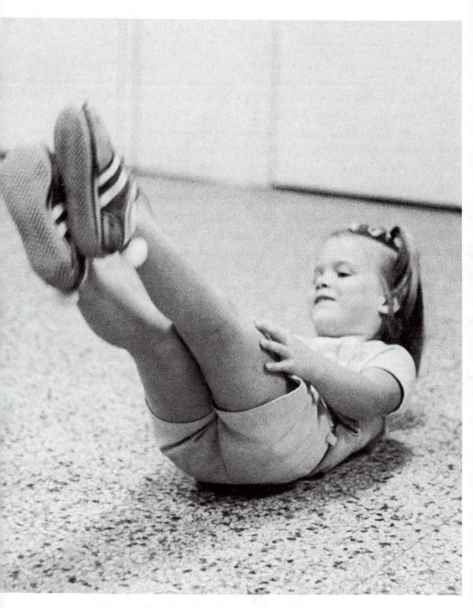

The children all get on the floor and rock like rocking horses until the signal is given to "jump off your rockers and gallop away!"

Rocky wanted to be a real live horse. What do real live horses do?

CHILDREN: Run. Walk.

TEACHER Do they do any work sometimes?

AARON: They run on tracks.

TEACHER: Oh yes, they go on race tracks. Did you ever see that? Did you see any horses when you went to the circus?

CHILDREN: We saw elephants . . . and clowns——and they were swinging on those two things. . . .

TEACHER: I know. You like to tell me all about what you saw at the circus. We talked about that last time. But did you see any horses?

CHILD: A lion jumped on the horse's back.

TEACHER: Do men ride on horses' backs sometimes?

CHILDREN: Yes.

TEACHER: And do you ever see horses on television? Do cowboys have horses? What do they do when they ride them?

CHILD #1: They go fast.

CHILD #2: They ride them when they go to rescue. . . .

TEACHER: Right, when they go to rescue people.

After this introduction to rocking horses, I generally tell the children the story of "Rocky," the toy rocking horse who wanted to be a "real, live horse and do what real, live horses do." Rocky rocked so hard that he finally jumped off his rockers and galloped away. First he met a policeman riding a big police horse. Rocky wanted to be a policeman's horse, but he wasn't *big* enough. He tried to pull a wagon like a farm horse, but he wasn't *strong* enough. He couldn't be a cowboy horse because he became frightened of the cows; he was not *brave* enough. He didn't run *fast* enough to be a race horse. Finally Rocky decided to go back to the store. He jumped back on his rockers and resumed his rocking happily.

Next I have the children act out this story in sequence, sometimes making up their own places for Rocky to visit. At the end I ask, "Why couldn't Rocky be a policeman's horse? A farmer's horse? A cowboy's horse? A race horse?" Each time the children respond with words that describe Rocky:

He was "little," not "big enough."
He was not "strong enough."
He was "afraid" and not "brave enough."
He was "too slow" and did not run "fast enough."

The concept of opposites is a rather advanced one for these four-year-olds, but through acting out the story, they were able to grasp it.

There are many familiar stories and classic fairy tales that children enjoy acting out. In my experience some of the children's favorites have been:

1. "The Sleeping Beauty"—the Tchaikovsky music has been put on record along with the narrative. Parts that are especially good for classroom scenes are

The townpeople coming to pay homage to the princess
The fairies making their wishes
The princess pricking her finger and falling asleep
The prince climbing the walls
The palace rejoicing at the wedding

2. "Cinderella"—the Prokovieff version has some good music for

The bickering of the ugly stepsisters
The appearing of the Fairy Godmother
Cinderella being transformed from ugliness to beauty

3. "The Gingerbread Man"—one class made up its own song for this:

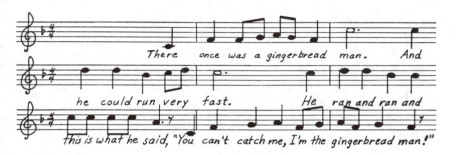

There once was a gingerbread man. And
he could run very fast. He ran and ran and
this is what he said, "You can't catch me, I'm the gingerbread man!"

4. "Hansel and Gretel"—there are many good scenes and music is available from the opera by Humperdinck. Children especially enjoy

Getting lost in the woods
Discovering the candy house

5. "Three Billy Goats Gruff" and "Three Bears" provide opportunities for contrasts in size of movements and in voices of the three animals. For younger groups, animal stories are excellent, because the movement quality of the animal involved can be interpreted.

Children soon learn to sense what stories are good for dramatization. With help from the teacher, a class can verbalize a set of criteria, such as the following:

1. The story must have action.
2. There must be changes in feeling.
3. It can have many characters, but only two or three should be involved in the action at the same time.
4. Characters with differing qualities make good dramatization.

Story dramatization has many functions in the primary grades. It involves the children, stimulates their thinking, and develops awarenesses—as do movement experiences of any type. In the early reading program of the lower grades, story dramatization serves the additional purpose of helping the teacher check the comprehension of beginning readers. The following account shows how this can be done:

A reading group in a second-grade class has just finished reading "Catching Tails."[7] "Can we act it out?" they ask. The teacher picks a chairperson to direct and assign roles, and the children are given a few minutes to plan on their own. They must consult their readers to see what answer the goat or the horse gave to the robin who wanted to know, "Why are you chasing your tail?" The children know that they need not use the exact words that are in the book, but they must be sure to act as the characters in the story did and to use words that convey the same ideas. When they are ready to begin, the teacher and the rest of the class prepare to be the audience.

The chairperson acts as the narrator and introduces the characters: "Jane is the kitten, Mark is the dog, Susan is the goat, Dorian is the horse, and Larry is the robin." The narrator starts reading the story as the kitten begins the action of chasing her tail. When the characters talk, the narrator stops, and the action is carried by the players acting the parts.

"Why are you chasing your tail?" says Mark, the dog.

"Because it is fun," answers Jane, the kitten.

"Then I will try it too," says the dog.

And so the action continues until all the animals have had their say. No books are used by the actors, although the narrator may serve as prompter if necessary. When the play is finished, the children may be a little dizzy, but they are certain that they

---

[7]Nancy K. Hosking, "Catching Tails," in *Friends and Neighbors*, Basic Reader—Second Grade (Chicago: Scott, Foresman, 1956), p. 121.

understood what each character in turn had to say about why he chased his tail!'

There are many stories in the readers most often used for primary grades that lend themselves readily to action. After the strain of sitting still and concentrating on small printed symbols, the children welcome the chance to move about, to stretch their muscles as well as their imaginations!

3 ಎ
Social Learning Through Movement

*T*he desks and chairs have been pushed back, and the children are forming a circle. The teacher is giving direction, holding a large Chinese gong in one hand, a soft tympany stick in the other. "Let's walk in a circle, taking big and fast steps when the gong is loud, and as the sounds fade away, let's make our steps slower and quieter. Go!" She strikes the gong, and its tones vibrate throughout the room. The children respond to the loud tone and run vigorously in a circle. As the sound dies down, they become quieter, and slower in their movement. As the last sound dies on the air, their movement stops.

"Look what happened to our circle! It's so small now," says Susan.

"Yes, it seemed right to close in together as the gong sound died away, and so you all did it together. When you are all concentrating hard, you can feel things together, without even talking about them, can't you?"

Group feeling is difficult to describe to a class, but they will sense it when it occurs. It happens sometimes with musical accompaniment, sometimes with narration, sometimes through unaccompanied movement. The quality shared need not be the same. It is important that the group is feeling together. It is a kind of artistic communication, mutually created.

If you believe that social studies begins with the relationships of children in a group, you will see why this description of the circle activity is used to introduce this chapter. It is an exercise that also develops a dynamic sense and relates quality of sound and movement.

Relationships Within a Group

It is recognized by modern educators that one of the purposes of a school program is to expose children to situations where they may function effectively as members of a group and where relationships to others can develop. Dancing is one of the activities well suited to this purpose. We often think of dancing as a social activity. Ballroom, square, and folk dancing are all means of socializing. Moving together with other people creates a friendly environment, and there is opportunity to get acquainted. But moving creatively in a classroom situation can do much more than this. Whether the children are working as individuals, in pairs, in small groups, or in large, they must be aware of what others are doing. They must relate to each other, although their movements may be different. There is a feeling of "oneness," where each individual is a part of a whole.

There are many social experiences that arise from the creative movement experiences of children in a classroom. A child may be given a chance to lead, to demonstrate a movement so that others may try it. Perhaps this is a child who might not have the opportunity for leadership in other areas of the program. Having the other children move with the leader provides reinforcement, and the others follow well, knowing that they may have the chance to lead at some other time.

Being "good audience" when another child or group has something to show is an important part of group living. Children need to learn to watch and become aware of the contributions of others. The evaluation sessions that follow must be fair and constructive.

The comments of the children as the group leader calls on them are beneficial both to the performers and to the observers.

When children work together on group studies, they have to create movements that blend and harmonize with those that others in the group are doing. Sometimes one child accompanies another's movements on a drum. Whatever the problem, there must be a give-and-take relationship within the group if it is to be worked out successfully. A more ambitious project might involve matters of organization concerned with staging, costuming, selling tickets, or issuing invitations. Each member of the class will find that his or her contribution is important. This is true in any group project where children work together. However, the challenging opportunities creative movement offers for this kind of development have been insufficiently explored.

Some readers may be saying, "Of course, the social relationships in a classroom are important, but are we really dealing with the *content* of the social studies program?" I believe that we are. Social studies cannot consist only in learning about geography, history, and politics. Relating to other individuals in a group is a type of social learning. Many adults join group dynamics or group therapy sessions to learn how to relate to others. Good social behavior is an important aspect of the curriculum and, like other skills, needs practice and reinforcement.

Teaching Safety

Safety is another important area of learning for young children. Social studies units in kindergarten and the primary grades frequently deal with topics related to health and safety. Here is a lesson using movement that developed from a discussion about street lights.

The teacher showed the children a stick with red, yellow, and green discs pasted to it. She asked the children what each color meant. Then they sang a song:

Red light, red light, what do you say?
I say STOP and stop right away.
Yellow light, yellow light, what do you mean?
I say WAIT until the light turns green.
Green light, green light, what do you say?
I say GO, but look both ways!

TEACHER: Let's play a game about stopping and going. Let's make a circle, and all go the same way. When Sandy points to the green light, we will all GO. We'll walk in time with my drum. When Sandy points to the yellow light, we will all walk slowly. When Sandy points to the red light, what will we do? STOP, that's right. Now we will listen to my drum, and we will watch Sandy as she points to the different colored lights. (Children do activity.)

Listen to the drum. Take one step every time you hear the drum. Good! I have another signal that means STOP. If I play my drum loudly, and then hold my stick up like this, that means STOP. Now let's try running when the drum goes fast. GO! And when the drum stops and I hold my stick up like this, you STOP. Good! You really know how to follow directions. Now we'll listen to the drum, and when the drum goes fast, we'll run, and when the drum goes slowly, we'll go slowly . . . and when the drum stops . . . we'll STOP.

Now, instead of using the drum, I am going to ask you to do what the light tells you to do. When I point to the green light, you may go. You may run if you like, but don't bump into people. When I point to the yellow light, what will you do?

CHILD: Slow down!

TEACHER: Yes, and then when I point to the red light, everyone must stop. Why is it important to follow directions, whether it's on a drum or by looking at colored lights?

CHILD #1:   So you don't get hurt!

CHILD #2:   So there are no accidents.

TEACHER: We need rules and signals to keep order on the street or in the classroom.

Study of safety rules can lead to discussion and study of various kinds of transportation. Children in nursery school and kindergarten love to move like cars, boats, and airplanes. Visiting in a kindergarten classroom in Japan, I was able to communicate with the children as we dramatized how I had arrived by plane, how I picked up my luggage, how I went on a bus to the hotel, and so on. The children did the action with me and understood just what I was telling them. Movement is a universal language!

Appreciating Cultural Diversity

An understanding of a culture, of a people, can be acquired through movement. When children move to African drums, they will experience the kind of feelings that Africans do. When third graders studying Indian tribes actually do a rain dance, they might understand better the Indian's desperate need for rain! In contrasting various ethnic dances, they come to understand differences in cultures and in the kinds of people who did these dances. Movement is another way of seeing things as other people might see them, a way to get into someone else's skin!

It has always been a source of amazement to me that children can sense the quality of music and will do spontaneous movements to various kinds of music that seem to fit that quality. Irish jigs result from lively selections like "The Irish Washerwoman." Greek music causes the children to bend their knees and move up and down, sometimes joining hands and weaving in and out of the circle. Even Kabuki music seems to result in Oriental types of

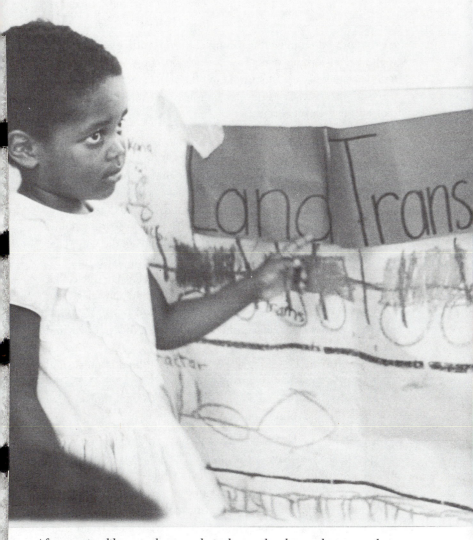

After moving like cars, boats and airplanes, the class makes a mural depicting different kinds of transportation.

movements when played to young children. Although they have
seen various ethnic dances on television, they surely are not
familiar enough with them to know the movements that go with
the kinds of music! Consider this sample of a lesson with four-year-
olds at a day care center:

TEACHER: I'm going to play some music, and I want you to make
              up a hopping dance. As you hop on one foot, see
              what you can do with the other foot. (Plays "Irish
              Washerwoman") Let's make a circle, and Aaron
              can go into the middle and show us his hopping
              dance. (Other children take turns) You didn't know
              that you knew how to do an Irish jig, did you? That
              was an Irish jig, ar d Irish people do that around St.
              Patrick's day. I see you made green shamrocks that
              are up on the wall. That is for St. Patrick's Day,
              too, isn't it?

              Let's do our hopping dance again. Now sit down and
              rest.

              Now I'm going to play a different kind of music and
              see how you can move to it. Move the way the
              music makes you feel. (Plays Greek music.) Do
              anything you like.

The children follow each other in a line, holding hands. When
Calypso music was played, the children became too excited and it
was necessary to stop the dancing for a while.

Possibly the best example I know of music as a means for
developing group and ethnic identity took place when I was in
Mississippi serving as consultant to a newly formed Head Start
class. At first it was difficult for shy, black children, brought to
town for the first time from their shacks along the delta, to listen
and respond to a northern white woman who had come to visit
their school. But when a song was sung that had a syncopated beat
("It's a Mighty Pretty Motion"), some of the children began to sway
in time to the music. One little girl said, "I knows a song like dat,"
and then proceeded to sing, "Give me more power, Lord."

As she sang, other children joined her, until soon they were all swaying and humming along with her. As she got louder, they moved more vigorously. As her singing became quieter, their movements slowed down. When she stopped, everyone stopped. It was a beautiful sight to see children responding so sensitively to each other, when they had been in a group for such a short period of time.

Music and movement can bring a group together, can help each member share and appreciate cultures other than their own, and can increase their pride in their own cultural heritage.

Movement Based on Work Themes

Work movements can do a great deal to break down the resistance of boys to creative movement. The problem has been lessened to some extent through the extensive use of male dancers on television, in movies, and in theater. Nevertheless, young boys will resist "dancing" unless it is called by another name. I like to say, "Move as if you are a farmer pitching hay" (or a baseball player). With a drum to set the rhythm, boys often create interesting movements greatly resembling dance!

A favorite game in kindergarten is based upon the following song:

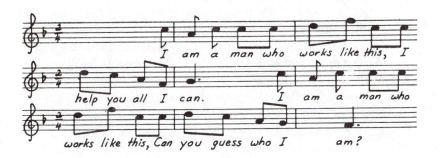

The children sing, while one does a work movement in time to the song. The class must guess what he or she is doing. Discussion follows in which children are made aware of the different kinds of work, and how the workers help us.

"Community helpers" is a common unit of social studies in primary grades. After some preliminary discussion and study, the class may be divided into groups where each is to make a report on a particular community helper. In addition to giving oral reports, each group might like to present dramatizations, showing the activities of firemen, policemen, nurses, or doctors, for instance. These can take the form of pure movement accompanied by drums or records, or they may be little plays in which dialogue is combined with movement to tell stories. The choice is left to the children in each group, and their own ideas for how to present what they have found out about their special "community helper" often reveal a great deal of what they have learned.

Classes in the primary grades often study ways of getting food, shelter, and clothing. The story of a product, such as wool, milk, or fruit, can be acted out so that the various stages of its processing is demonstrated to the class. This is a lively way of presenting material that is being studied, and sometimes it grows into something more than a simple movement study. The resultant product may have the artistic qualities of a dance.

One third grade class combined some of these movements into a group dance. One group of children did a variety of "factory movements," creating a staccato, mechanical effect. Another group used the best of the improvised movements relating to a farm. The groups alternated, first factory workers moving, then farm workers, then factory again, and so on. Other children provided suitable accompaniment on rhythm instruments, while one child improvised a theme for each at the piano. The best movements were selected, exaggerated, and set in sequence. The dance may not have been an artistic achievement, but the experience of re-creating movements involved in various types of production was valuable to the children. For some, it increased understanding of the social studies unit studied. It was satisfying for all to use their new knowledge to create something of their own that had quality and that unified some of their experiences.

Dramatizing History Studies

Lessons in social living sometimes evolve without previous inducement by the teacher. On the day before Lincoln's Birthday, a second grade class decided to enact some scenes from Lincoln's life. Selections of incidents were made from a story the teacher had read. The class was divided into four groups, and four scenes were planned. Two of them proved to be of special interest, not only because of what they told of Lincoln's life, but because of the revealing portrayal of character that two of the "Lincolns" showed in their acting.

Ian portrayed Lincoln as the storekeeper who walked ten miles to return the penny that he owed to a customer.

"Here is your penny," said Ian to Susan who was the customer. "I walked ten miles to give it to you. I am very honest."

The class sensed that this was not how Lincoln would have behaved. There was some discussion about "bragging." The children agreed that a great man like Lincoln would not brag about himself. This was more than an incident in history that Ian had enacted. He was a braggart who had created a Lincoln in his own image! Perhaps he learned about more than Lincoln from his portrayal.

Skippy portrayed Lincoln "freeing the slaves." The scene was an imaginary one in which Lincoln visited a plantation and saw some slaves working and being mistreated by the owner. Immediately Skippy began an argument. "You can't treat those people that way! They are just as good as you! If you don't stop that, I'll beat you up!"

Skippy is a scrapper who is quick to challenge others on the playground as well as in a play! His "Lincoln" surprised no one, and they were quick to point out that the real Lincoln would not have handled the situation in quite the same way.

Historical events are remembered by children when they have been dramatized. Elementary school children can not be expected to learn all the facts about their government, their country's history, or that of other countries. What is important is that they gain knowledge of the society in which they live and respect for their country's great heritage, and that they develop understandings of the roles they are to play in that society and in the preservation and re-creation of that heritage. The emphasis must be upon spiritual and moral values. These can be heightened when the children are involved in creative movement, and when the quality of the movement is emphasized.

A fifth-grade group was studying a unit on early American life. The children had worked through the landing of the Pilgrims at Plymouth Rock in movement. This was done to music, with an occasional narration. The excitement, the thrill of discovery, the hope and courage of these people were directly experienced by the children as they portrayed their roles. This was not simply the dramatization of a scene or pantomime; there were qualities of artistic dance in this study. There was rhythmic pattern, an apparent form, and most of all, there was projection of emotion through bodily movement.

The same unit on early American life was the subject for a social studies unit in another class. In this group, the children had had less exposure to creative-movement activity, and some boys resisted sincere participation. They were quick to use the time for silliness and high jinks.

The teacher gave them a special assignment. They were to find out how the first settlers built their homes, what equipment they used, what materials, and how they worked. They were sent to the library, while the rest of the class worked on movement studies.

They returned to the class later, anxious to communicate what they had found. Their silliness had left them, and they were involved and eager now. The teacher said, "Do you think you could show us how they worked, while you tell about it?" Two boys worked at sawing a tree, two others made mortar by pushing heavy sticks around a central container, heavy logs were carried by two more. The teacher used her drum to set a time, and soon all of these work movements were synchronized into a single rhythm. The resultant movement study was used as one scene in the saga of early American life presented later at an assembly program by this class.

Understanding Forms of Government

An interesting experiment was tried in one sixth-grade class. The children had done movement studies throughout the term and were familiar with the pattern of working in groups, planning their ideas, and presenting them to others. The teacher picked two capable chairpersons one day and called them aside for some preliminary discussion.

"I know that you both know how to be good chairpersons," she said. "You know how to take suggestions from members of your group and to put them together so that the best ideas are worked into your play. You know that the more you let each member contribute, the better the group will work together. I'd like to try a little experiment this morning, to show the class that this is true.

"Ned, I would like you to be the best chairman you know how to be. Let everyone have a part in making the play. Let the group help you decide who should play each part. Vote on things if there is disagreement. Try to give everyone something important to do.

"Barbara, I'd like to see if you could act differently, just for today. You select the story, and tell each member of the group what to do. Be as bossy as you can be. Do not let anyone else have a chance to give an opinion. Let's see what happens."

Ned and Barbara enjoyed the secret that the teacher had entrusted to them, and they carried off their roles well. Ned's group went off to one side of the room and proceeded to plan. There was lively discussion, some noisy enthusiastic voices raised, and then a quieting down as each member began to work on his or her own part. They had chosen a story from a reader, and they went to the book to check details. Some took notes, others worked with construction paper designing props. The chairman circulated around making suggestions and seeing that each member was busy.

Barbara selected a story she knew but one that was unfamiliar to the others in her group. She was trying to tell it to them, but already there were voices raised in protest. The children ran to the teacher's desk, complaining that "Barbara is unfair." "She won't listen to anybody." "She won't let us talk!" The teacher shrugged and told them they must do as their chairwoman tells them.

There was some grumbling, but the children sullenly complied. When it was time to show each other what they had done, Ned's group performed with enthusiasm and both performers and audience enjoyed it. Barbara had actually devised a better play, but her group was listless in its performance. Some had dropped out and would not take any part in it. Barbara was the narrator, and often she had to tell the performers what to do in order to keep the action going. The audience was quick to sense this and to comment about it during the discussion that followed.

"Can I tell them now?" Barbara asked. "I don't want everyone to think I'm really that bossy!"

The secret was told, and the class thought it was a great joke. But the teacher was quick to point out the significance of the experiment. A discussion ensued about democratic versus autocratic methods. Observations were made about the way people behave under each system. Parallels were drawn to governments in other countries. "Dictatorship," "fascism," and "parliamentary procedure" were defined and clarified. A lesson in social studies evolved that would not be easily forgotten.

Geography Through Movement

In today's school program, geography is often integrated with other aspects of the social studies unit. Study of products of a country would include where these products came from, and why such an area was well suited for the production of a particular item. Creative movement studies can be related to geography as well as to other social studies areas.

A fourth-grade class began a unit with the question, "How do rivers affect the life of the people who live near them?" They investigated various rivers, studying the rivers' sources and the life of the people in those mountain areas. They traced the river on the map and discovered the industries that flourished along the way. They found the big cities at the mouth of each river and accounted for their existence there.

A culminating program for the study of rivers included a dramatization called "Life of the River." Action began with a babbling brook, high in a mountain. A poem was the accompaniment for the movement of some children representing the brook. The movement continued in more subdued fashion as animals of the forest came to drink from the brook. Loggers chopped down trees, and floated them down the river to the sawmill. As the brook became a slow, moving river wending its way through farm land, other children represented the farmers at work. The life of the city at the mouth of the river was represented by factory workers, by hustle and bustle, by large boats and tugs in the harbor. The dance ended when the river became part of the huge ocean, with most of the class representing the waving motions of the sea. A few sea-gulls, represented by other children, circled about as the only signs of life.

This was a large undertaking that involved language arts (poems), music (rhythmic accompaniment), and art (scenery), as well as all the various aspects of social studies. Perhaps we can say that no subject can be completely isolated from others, either in the classroom or in life. Just as geography is related to the life of the people in the locale studied, so creative movement relates many areas of learning, pointing up relationships among them and integrating them all into a meaningful whole.

4 ﷼

Movement as an Aid in Mastering Number Concepts

*C*hildren react to music; they move to rhythm. They don't feel they are learning arithmetic, but there is an incidental learning going on. If teachers are aware of this relationship, they can make use of it to clarify number concepts. A musician needs a number system to count out the rhythm of music. The young child has a strong sense of rhythm and can keep time to intricate rhythms long before knowing how to "count it out." The musician uses numbers to help clarify rhythm; the child, conversely, can use rhythm to clarify number concepts.

Reading Rhythms

Children as young as three years of age are able to identify rhythmic patterns and can even learn to "read" rhythms when symbols have been established to represent the sounds. In developing this facility, we began by having a group of three-year-olds play the rhythms of their names on drums. We then added the cymbal on the accent. Thus, for "Erin Weiss," we played two short beats and the cymbal for the last name. Next I asked the children to move around in a circle, taking two short steps and a jump as we chanted, "Erin *Weiss*, Erin *Weiss*, Erin *Weiss*." We decided to write this on the blackboard in the following way:

| | * | | * | | *

We developed similar sequences of symbols for the other children's names. At a session a week later these three-year-olds were able to recognize the written symbols that stood for their names. Each child could point to his or her name on the blackboard, could play it on the drum, and could walk in time to the rhythm that was played.

At the four-year-old level, children can learn to count as they play their rhythm instruments and move in time to the beats. Suppose we want them to understand the meaning of "four." The teacher plays four beats on the drum, and the children count in time. Frequently they will continue to count "one, two, three, four, five, six . . ." until the teacher makes it clear that they are to count only the beats on the drum, and to stop counting when the drum stops playing. When the children have done this successfully, they have established one-to-one correspondence through the auditory channel.

The children can then make combinations that add up to four. They may take two walking steps and two jumps. The drums can be played for the walking and the cymbals for the jumps. Thus, we have | | * * making four beats all together. Four-year-olds begin to understand that two walks and two jumps add up to four beats.

Counting with the Rhythm Orchestra

Counting beats can be developed further by having four-year-olds play in a rhythm orchestra where each instrument takes a different part to play. The teacher might introduce this activity in the following way:

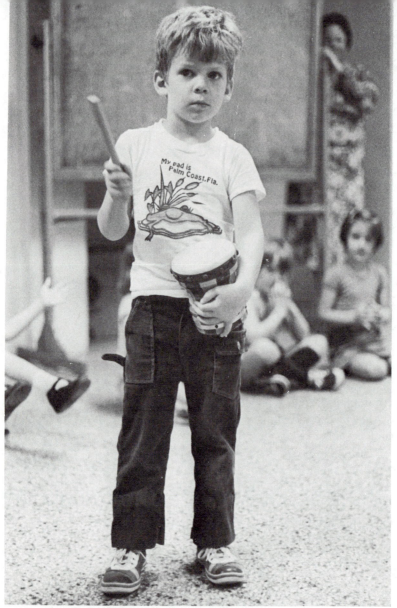

"Can you make the drum say your name?" Each beat stands for a syllable. Auditory discrimination is developed as each child learns to play and identify his or her own name.

TEACHER: Do you know what is going to happen today? Do you know how I always play drum talk for you? Well, today you are going to make the drum talk. You are going to follow directions and you're going to make some of your own directions for other people to follow. What does it mean when the leader does this (holding stick up in air)?

CHILDREN: Stop!

TEACHER: And when I give you an instrument to play (I have all these instruments over here), and when I put my stick up in the air that means stop playing. Did you ever see an orchestra with a conductor on television? When the conductor holds a stick up, everyone stops playing and waits for the next signal. Sit in a circle on the edge of the rug, close your eyes, and I will put an instrument down behind you. Don't look, keep your eyes closed. (Distributes instruments by type.) Now everyone turn around and pick up the instrument that is behind you. You may try it to see how it sounds. (Holds stick up.) What does it mean when I put my stick up? (Repeat playing and stopping.) When you play a drum, you should hold it up so it doesn't touch anything, and make the stick bounce off the drum. If it has a skin like this, we'll call it a drum. One, two, three, four, five people have drums. We'll call these things sticks because they are made out of wood. If you have a stick, put your hand in the air. When you hear an orchestra or a band, does everyone play the same thing? No, they play different things—sometimes the drums play, sometimes the sticks play, sometimes the bells play, and sometimes the cymbals play. Let me hear just the drums play. Let me hear the sticks play. Now let me hear the bells

play. We'll call the triangles bells too, so they can
play when the bells play. Let me hear the cymbals
play. Now listen. We will play, "Are you sleeping,
Brother John?" just like an orchestra might play it:

Are you sleeping Are you sleeping	*Drums play on each beat as children sing.*
Brother John? Brother John?	*Sticks play on each beat as children sing.*
Morning bells are ringing Morning bells are ringing	*Bells play on each beat (twice as fast).*
Ding Dong Ding Ding Dong Ding	*Cymbals play.*

After the children have learned to orchestrate the song, with
different instruments playing different parts, they may learn to
count what they have played. At the next session, the teacher
might follow the playing of "Brother John" with a counting exercise:

TEACHER: Now that we have played, "Are you sleeping," who
             can tell me how many times we beat the drum
             while we sang that?

CHILDREN: Four

TEACHER: That's right. "Are you sleep—ing" has four beats. And
             if we play it again, how many beats does that make?

CHILDREN: five . . . six.

TEACHER: No, you are guessing. Let's count.

Are you sleep—ing
1   2   3   4
Are you sleep——ing
5   6   7   8

You see, if we have four two times, that makes eight.

If the children learn to count the beats accurately, they can then go on to discover what happens when the beats are twice as fast, as in, "Morning bells are ringing." This can be counted as, "one and two and three, four." If the children understand this, they can begin to notate the rhythm, using short and long lines, as explained later in this chapter.

Identifying Shapes

Learning to identify shapes is an important skill for three- and four-year-olds. They need the visual discrimination involved in recognizing circles, squares, and triangles in order to see differences in letters of the alphabet. Knowing shapes is also related to simple geometry and to classification. These are mathematical concepts necessary for all later learning in that discipline. Making shapes with their bodies is one way to reinforce knowledge about shapes. Here is a transcript from part of a movement session with four-year-olds:

TEACHER: Let's see you take enough space and not touch anyone. Can you make a circle with your arms. Go around your body. That makes you want to turn around, doesn't it? How else can you make a circle? Look at Amond's circle. He is making a very little one just with his fingers. Look at this, I can draw a circle on the floor with my foot.

CHILD #1:   I can make one!

CHILD #2:   I'm going to make a little circle.

TEACHER: Now make a circle anyway you like. Aaron has a circle with his arms over his head. Make your arms round. Let's see if you can do this. Make a circle with your arms in front, now up over your head, now bring your arms out to the side, and then down (doing balletic port de bras). O.K. I have some pictures that you have made, and I'm going to ask you to tell me what shapes you see. Yes, that's a triangle. Can you make a triangle with your arms? Look, here's a triangle.

CHILD #3:   See? I can make a triangle.

TEACHER: Good. Do you see two triangles when Jesse puts his hands on his hips? Take a partner and see if you can make a square. O.K. I'm going to make a sound on my drum, and you're going to make a shape, and then I'm going to guess what shape it is. (Children make different shapes, and the teacher comments on each.)

Numerals as Floor Patterns

Learning to write numerals requires a spacial awareness that can be developed through movement. In a kindergarten or first-grade classroom, children can learn the shapes of numerals as they trace them in movement.

The numeral "3" often confuses children. They have a tendency to write it backwards. At a rhythms session, the class might draw a large 3 on the floor in chalk. Now instead of walking in a circle in time to the drum, the children might follow the shape of the 3, starting at the top, and coming across the room in two big curves. They might take the feel of the curve into their bodies as they go. They might take the first loop walking forward, and the second loop walking backward. They might make an accent in their rhythm as they change directions in the middle. Some interesting movement patterns develop as the children do this.

One child at a time may take a turn, perhaps erasing the

numeral on the floor and trying other numerals. The group that is watching may try to guess what numeral is being done.

The shape of the floor pattern is emphasized, and the children feel the shape as they move through it. A curve has a different feeling from a straight line, and they will naturally lean in the direction of the curve as they go. This exercise stimulates children to use more interesting arrangements in their use of space. Although it does not relate to number concept, it is practice in the recognition of number symbols, and it contributes to their learning in arithmetic.

Components of Numbers—Addition and Subtraction

The members of a first-grade class take their rhythm instruments one day, and begin to make a percussion orchestra. Some children have drums, some have tone blocks, some triangles, and two boys are given the cymbals.

The teacher begins the class by asking the children to keep time with the drum. The teacher plays an even beat, varying the tempo. The children must watch and listen carefully to stay with the beat. They must concentrate, and soon the teacher senses their complete attention.

"Let's have each group of instruments play something different," the teacher says. "The cymbals are playing on 'one'; what would the drums like to play?" The drum players decide to play on "two, three, and four." They would pause on "one," while the cymbals play alone.

"Can the blocks play something different, and still keep time with the rest of us?" Steven begins a rhythm that divides the third beat in half. "Fine! The blocks will play 'three-and-four,' as Steven is doing. Do not play on 'one' and 'two,' so that we can hear the other instruments, then. If you hit the air with your sticks on those beats, you will be able to keep the rhythm." The children practice a while with the teacher's help. They try their parts alone, and then with the other instruments.

"Now what would the triangles like to play?" Susan had already begun to play every other beat, hitting the air on the silent ones in between. "Let's do what Susan is doing:"

1	2	3	4
Play	Hit the air	Play	Hit the air

The teacher does it with the triangle group until they feel secure, then they try it with the whole orchestra.

Now each group of instruments is playing a different rhythm while they count to four. The teacher selects some children to move to it. They may relate to one group of instruments, moving only on the beats played by them, or they may move freely, as the rhythm of the whole orchestra makes them feel. Interesting patterns in movement result.

The children enjoy moving about the room, while others play. They take turns, moving and playing, all the while keeping the various combinations of four going in the orchestra.

"Now we will write down what we have done on the chalkboard," the teacher says. "See how many different ways we have found to make four?"

Instrument	What Was Played				Combination of 4
Cymbals	1	2	3	4	$1+3=4$
	Play	Pause	Pause	Pause	
Drums	1	2	3	4	$3+1=4$
	Pause	Play	Play	Play	
Blocks	1	2	3 and 4		$2+\frac{1}{2}+\frac{1}{2}+1=4$
	Pause	Pause	Play		
Triangles	1	2	3	4	$2+2=4$
	Play	Pause	Play	Pause	

Explaining what was written on the board, the teacher might say:

"You see, the cymbals played one beat and were silent for three others. The drums did just the opposite. The blocks were silent for two beats, and then they played two halves on 'three' and a whole one on 'four.' The triangles played every other beat, so they played twice and were silent twice."

This may look very complicated in writing, but the children understand it once they have done it. They may try making up their own symbols for recording what they have played. The need for symbolic representation becomes clear if they decide they want to play the same arrangement another time:

Instrument and Code	Key
Cymbals: | – – –	| = whole beat
Drums: – | | |	ı = half beat
Blocks: – – ı ı |	– = pause
Triangles: | – | –	

The children in the first-grade class became aware of "four-ness," and this awareness reached them through several sensory channels at the same time. They heard the rhythm. They saw the movement and later the symbols representing the rhythms written on the board. They sensed kinesthetically through moving themselves.

Similar studies could be worked around numbers other than four. The fact that music is often grouped into counts of four does not mean that we cannot use five, six, or seven as a basis for making up rhythm combinations with children. Different groupings of beats can be made up of loud and soft, of alternating percussion sounds, or of pauses and beats. Various ways of contrasting beats can be used, so that the components of any number that the children are studying can be made clear to them.

Another way of developing awareness of the different combinations making up a given number is to allow the children to move about the room, forming various *groupings* as in a square dance.

The teacher might take the number seven, for example, and have a pianist or a phonograph playing a lively square dance tune, such as "Skip to my Lou." The dance begins with seven boys and girls skipping in one large circle, holding hands. The music stops. They must break into smaller groups, at the same time calling out the combinations, such as "four and three." The music starts, and they skip again. When the music stops, they must form new groupings, such as "three, two, and two"; and so on until all possible combinations of seven have been tried. This idea could be worked out in a more formal movement study as well.

It is possible to use different groupings, as described above, in conjunction with various themes that have been discussed, such as a farm theme. A teacher might select three movements that the children have done depicting work on the farm. The group "pitching hay" might take one corner of the room. The "planters" might be on the floor in the center of the room. Another group might be "picking apples" in a third section of the room. Nine children have been chosen, and they may do any one of these three activities.

The other children in the class are seated at the side, and they are to write down on pieces of paper the combinations that they see in the groupings of children who are performing. The children decide on three even groups to start, each group having three members. The music starts (any lively Western music may be used). The children begin their action in time to the music. A beat on the drum is the signal to change groups. The children have been told to make the transition smoothly, as if each of the "farmers" decided to do a different chore. It is important not to destroy the mood created in order to emphasize number relationships.

The music goes on, and at appropriate places the teacher sounds the drum for the groups to change. Some "farmers" who were "planting" move slowly over to the "apple orchard" and start "picking." One of these "pickers" decides to "pitch hay." Thus, new groupings are formed, and the movement goes on. The movement study has become more interesting because of these changes in pattern.

The children who are watching write down the new combinations they see. There is to be no talking until the dance is finished. Both the performers and the audience respect this rule. When the music comes to an end, the dancers take their seats, and the discussion begins. The children and the teacher comment about the quality of the movement, and the way it was performed. Then, one observer is asked to read her list of combinations that she saw. The teacher writes it on the board:

Pitching Hay		Planting		Picking Apples		Total
3	+	3	+	3	=	9
4	+	1	+	4	=	9
5	+	4	+	0	=	9
6	+	0	+	3	=	9

The children compare their lists with what has been put on the board.

Fractions Through Rhythm

To demonstrate how fractions can be taught through movement, let's look at a third-grade class where the children are familiar with movement, have worked with rhythm instruments, and have made and orchestrated rhythms of their own. They discussed fractions in the arithmetic lesson this morning. Now they are starting a rhythms session:

"Girls make a circle with your left shoulder to the center, and walk in the line of direction in time to the drum. Good! Keep it nice and even, now." The teacher's drum is playing an even walking beat.

"Can one of the boys go around in the other direction, taking two steps to the girls' one? Yes, you must go twice as fast. Mark, you try it. No, that is not right because one of your steps takes longer than the other." Mark had begun to run with an uneven (long, short) rhythm. "Walter, you try it. Remember that you are dividing the girls' time in half. Both halves must be the same size." Walter does it correctly, and all the boys are asked to join in the outside circle, going clockwise.

When the children feel secure in the rhythm of each group, the teacher suggests that they count the number of steps. "We'll start with the girls taking four slow walking steps. If the boys divide this beat in half, how many steps would they take?"

After the children have responded with the correct number of eight, and have tried it moving in the circle and counting, the teacher might draw some comparisons with their previous discussion of fractions. "Remember the pie we drew on the board this morning? When each quarter was divided into half again, we had eight pieces, didn't we? Each piece is one eighth of the whole circle. The boys have been running to eighth notes while the girls walked to quarter notes."

The children try the exercise in reverse, that is, the boys beginning with running steps first, and the girls finding the tempo that takes one step to every two of the boys. They switch roles. They try other numbers. They find that this can be done with only even numbers, so they try six, eight, ten, and twelve, dividing them in half, then doubling them, exploring relationships in various ways.

A more difficult feat is to divide a beat into thirds. If the children have learned to do a waltz, they will soon be able to count one, two, three, keeping the duration even although the first beat is stronger. Now while one group walks slowly on the strong beat, the other group runs a triplet, dividing the whole beat into thirds. They can find out in a way similar to that described above that four walking beats divided into thirds gives twelve running beats, and so forth.

Rhythm Helps in Multiplication

Rhythm instruments, and moving in time to them, can help with many other aspects of number work.

In the primary grades, children learn to count by twos, threes, fours, and fives, in preparation for multiplying. Suppose a class needed drill in counting in this way. Asking one child after another to stand up and count will be boring to the rest of the class. But suppose, while the one child is counting by twos, half of the class plays drums, and the other half moves in a circle in time to the beat. To develop the concept, the student who is counting should begin counting by ones, accenting the even numbers with his or her voice:

1 2 3 4 5 6 7 8 9 10 11 12

Those who have rhythm instruments might play in this way:

   Drums, play on every beat

   Blocks, play only on even numbers

or:

   Drums, play on odd numbers

   Blocks, play on even numbers

Of course, the instruments may be interchanged, or others substituted or added. The child who is counting may now try counting only even numbers aloud. The instruments will help a student who has been having difficulty. (The teacher will have chosen a child to do this who needs help in understanding.)

The children who are moving in the circle will take light steps on the odd numbers and heavy steps on the even numbers. Soon they will begin to count the even numbers (those accented) aloud as they move in time.

A similar plan can be followed for counting by threes, fours, and fives:

1 2 3 4 5 6 7 8 9 10 11 12
1 2 3 4 5 6 7 8 9 10 11 12 13 14 15 16
1 2 3 4 5 6 7 8 9 10 11 12 13 14 15

There are ways of varying this learning experience. Suppose we are counting by fives. A strong crash on the cymbal can be used for every fifth beat. The children who are walking in time would then take light steps for one, two, three, four and a jump or strong accented movement on the fifth.

It might be tried standing in one place on the floor. The light beats are slow, sustained movements; the cymbal on the fifth beat is a strong accented movement, possibly with a change in direction. An arm swing might then be:

1 2 3 4 5 6 7 8 9

Arms slowly raised to the left.   Change direction moving arm
                                    in arc to the opposite side.

On ten the swing is reversed again, and so on. The children will do well in making their own movements to fit these rhythmic patterns. They should change places, so that those who are moving have a turn with the instruments, and those playing instruments have a turn moving. They should, after a while, count only the fifth (accented) beat aloud, while the pause (one, two, three, four) is felt in their bodies. Their rhythmic sense will thus be helping them to feel the multiples of five.

Examples have been given of the use of movement to develop numerical understanding related to adding, subtracting, multiplying, and dividing. I am not claiming that movement and rhythm should be the sole approach to the development of number concept. But learning arithmetic need not be a sedentary or static part of the school curriculum. It can be active, stimulating, and meaningful. Teachers can use movement and rhythm in such a way that the interest of children will be directed toward arithmetic learning itself. Through movement, we can develop a conscious awareness of number relations and their significance.

5 ❧
Movement in the
Science Program

With the advent of television and the space age, children's horizons have broadened considerably. They know about space stations and satellites. They want to know how these things work. They ask questions that are difficult for teachers to answer in terms that are meaningful.

Teachers must find ways to make these difficult concepts understandable. They may use charts, models, and experiments. But if children are encouraged to "identify" with what they see outside themselves, another avenue of understanding is opened. A four- or five-year-old boy may be seen making believe that he is the sun. He hides behind a chair, comes up slowly, moves across the room with arms outstretched, and sinks behind a "mountain," which is another chair.

Imaginative play helps the very young child to understand more about his world. Using the same principle of "identification," the teacher can help the child in the elementary grades to understand some of the basic concepts of science.

Living Things

The young child identifies with what he observes in nature. Notice, in the picture on page 76, the way in which the little girl imitates the movement of the duck that she is observing.

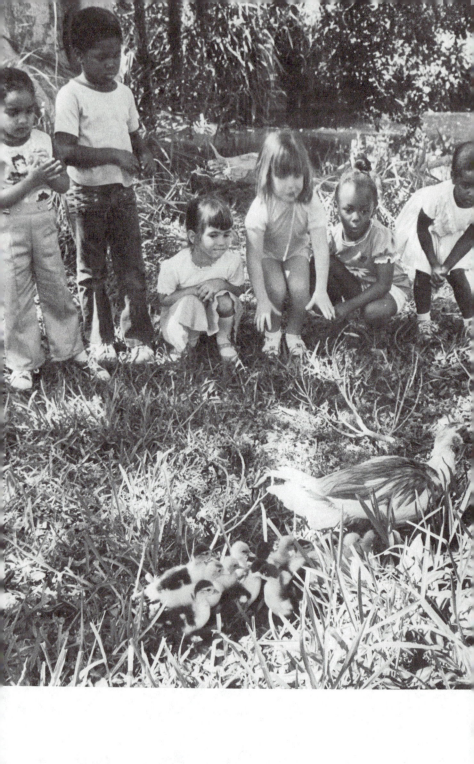

Observation of nature—of animal and plant life—starts very early in a child's experience. Two-year-olds are fascinated by the antics of dogs and cats. A visit to a zoo is exciting to nursery school or kindergarten children. Their awareness of what they have seen is heightened if they have a chance, in their rhythmic play, to imitate the animals they have observed.

"Today we will pretend that we are at the zoo," the kindergarten teacher says, and the children respond enthusiastically. "Teddy, what do you want to be?"

"I'll be a lion," says Teddy.

"All right, the lion cage is in that corner." The teacher indicates a section of the room. Other children choose to be bears, elephants, giraffes, monkeys, and seals, and they are assigned areas of space in which to move. Some children might care to be the visitors to the zoo. They join the teacher strolling about and viewing the "animals." Rhythm records that suggest animal movements might be used for accompaniment, but this time the teacher is using a drum and keeping time for each "animal" as their cages are visited.

"Look at those seals pulling themselves along on their stomachs with their flippers. Now they are diving into the water. "Paul," the teacher addresses a boy who has not participated, "You be the caretaker who feeds them some fish. Let's see how they stretch their spines to catch them."

The teacher is suggesting some of the action, calling attention to some good movements, and providing continuity and order to the action. The teacher does not show the children how to do the movements. The stereotyped "elephant walk" and "duck waddle" have no place here. The children's ideas in movement are better than this. All the teacher is doing is calling attention to some of the

Young children identify with what they observe in nature. Notice the way in which the little girl in the middle imitates the movement of the duck she is observing.

qualities and actions of the animals that the children might have observed at the zoo. They become aware of characteristics that they had not consciously observed as they "move like" the animals they saw.

All kinds of animals are fun to do in movement. An imaginary visit to a farm or woods evokes interesting interpretations of chickens, turkeys, ducks, rabbits, and frogs. Many stories in the readers for the first and second grades tell about animals. Acting these out makes the stories "come alive" for the children, but the action can also focus attention on the qualities of the animals themselves.

"Tom didn't jump like a frog," Nancy said, when Tom had finished his portrayal of an animal story from the second-grade reader. "A frog pushes off with his back legs like this, and he keeps his front legs in between."

Story dramatization can sharpen powers of observation. The ability to observe keenly is a prime requisite of a scientist.

Nursery or kindergarten children love to play a game in which one child goes into the middle of a circle and acts like an animal. The other children try to guess what animal it is.

Sometimes the teacher may suggest the action by telling a riddle. The children guess the animal referred to and then do the action. Some riddles that may be used for this activity include:

1. They prowl back and forth in their cages.
   They raise up their heads when they roar.
   Answer: Lions and tigers

2. They waddle.
   They swim in a pond.
   They dip their heads to get a worm.
   Answer: Ducks and geese

3. They have long heavy tails that drag.
   They catch fish in their mouths.
   Sometimes they lie on their back and flap their flippers.
   Answer: Seals

Poems often suggest the action of animals. A popular one with children is:

> Creepy, crawly, wiggly, squiggly caterpillar funny,
> You will be a butterfly, when the days are sunny!
> Winging, flinging, dancing, singing
> Butterfly, so yellow,
> You were once a caterpillar,
> Creepy, crawly fellow!

A four-year-old, after acting out this poem, proceeded to tell the class the entire story of metamorphosis. Later, the children drew pictures of caterpillars and butterflies, and the teacher made an "experience chart" explaining the process in the children's own words.

It was through movement that these young children began to understand a complicated process in nature. Imaginative play helps very young children comprehend more about their surroundings. Using the same process of identification, teachers can help older children understand some basic concepts in science.

Force, Motion, and Machines

"What makes a rocket go?" asks a first-grader. Even a teacher who was an engineer would have difficulty explaining the mechanism. But the principle of action-reaction can be demonstrated to the class through movement.

The children sit on the floor in pairs with legs outstretched, feet touching, and holding hands. As one pushes forward, the other pulls back. Then the one who has been pulling starts pushing, and the roles are thus reversed. The force exerted by each is the same, but in the opposite direction. "Every action force has an equal and opposite reaction force."

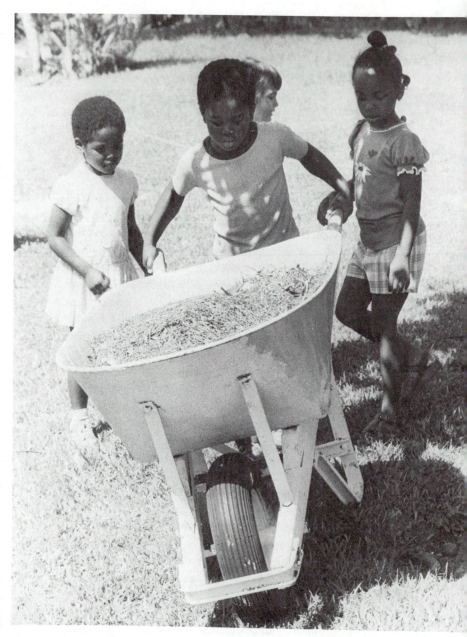

Pushing and balancing are experienced as children use a wheelbarrow.

A rocket works on this principle. It pushes against its launching platform with terrific force; then, when the rocket is released—since the platform can not be pushed down—the same force works in the opposite direction and sends the rocket up into space.

"You use the same principle when you ride on a scooter," the teacher says. "You push the ground backward with your foot; the ground does not move, so the scooter goes forward. Let's all pretend we are riding scooters, and you will see what I mean."

The principle of action-reaction can be developed further in movement study. Without really touching each other, two children can work together to demonstrate how one reacts to the force of the other's movement. They can find different ways to exert the force, that is, to push. The second child reacts with movements that are equal in force, but in the opposite direction. Some interesting movement patterns result.

A fourth-grade class has been studying simple machines and how they work. They are working in pairs now, pushing and pulling, reacting physically to the degree of intensity of their partners' movements.

"What kind of machine uses the principle of action-reaction?" the teacher asks.

"Rowing a boat works something like that, doesn't it?" Susan volunteers. "As we push forward, the boat goes backward."

"Yes," Frank says. "And the harder we push the faster it goes. Like this!"

"Yes," the teacher says. "We can call the oars a kind of simple machine."

"Now let's see how a pulley works," the teacher suggests. "One of you be at the end of the rope that pulls. The other be the object that is pulled. You don't have to touch each other—just react to your partner's movement."

Levers and screws are demonstrated in a similar way. If the children understand the action of these simple machines, they will enjoy the challenge of translating them into movement. For others who might not have grasped the ideas from discussion, the live demonstration makes the concept clear. Later, perhaps, the children might be made aware of the dance qualities of rhythm, dynamics, levels, and pattern that can result from such movement exploration. Combinations can be built into a group dance that not only demonstrates what has been learned, but becomes an aesthetic experience as well.

Other laws of motion can be readily demonstrated through movement. The game of "statues" often played on the playground illustrates the principle of centrifugal force. A girl holds one hand of a boy and spins him around several times. When she lets go, the boy flys off into "space" and must remain in the position he stops in. The girl then spins each member of the class and chooses the best "statue" to have a turn as the spinner. Children that participate in this activity to learn about centrifugal force can more easily relate this principle to other areas where it functions.

Units on transportation lend themselves readily to dramatization. Children love to simulate the motion of a train, moving arms in circular patterns to represent the wheels, starting off slowly and building speed as they go. Showing the various types of boats in a harbor makes an interesting movement study. The movement of tugboats, motorboats, and large ocean liners can be portrayed, and the differences in quality of movement among them can be sensed as the children move.

An electrical circuit can be demonstrated by asking children to hold hands in a line. An "impulse," in this case, a simple body movement, passes along from one child to another along the length of the line. A "broken circuit" occurs when one child steps out of the line. Then the "impulse" or movement stops at this point and does not travel to the end. A "closed circuit" can end with the hitting of a bell or drum, by the last child. The "open circuit" has no culminating sound.

"Close" and "open" are also words that represent the action of our joints. One of the ways we have to explore movement is a warm-up stretch in which the children are asked to "close in all together," and then "open up and stretch." They sit on the floor to begin, knees to chest and arms pulled in close to the body. As they "open out," they stretch legs and arms to the side and straighten their spines. On a sharp drum beat, they return to the original position.

A first-grader once commented, "My mother has chairs that do this." That led to a discussion on the action of hinges and how our own bodies have "hinges" at the elbow, knee, for example, that allow us to "close" and "open" in the same way. From this time on, the children insisted on calling this exercise "Folding Chairs." They experimented with using their bodies to make other folding and opening movements, in standing position, on knees, and lying down. Expansive movements have a very different feeling from those of contraction. Children were asked what kind of feeling they get when they reach out, and how they feel when they pull in. They did improvisations on this, some with story ideas and some that were just mood pictures. Things in nature that "open" and "close," such as a turtle coming out of and going into its shell or a moth emerging from its cocoon, make use of these movements.

Movement in Space

Interest in space today makes it mandatory that some study of astronomy take place in the elementary grades and movement can be helpful in clarifying the complexities in this subject. One science supervisor says she cannot explain the difference between rotation and revolution to sixth-graders without showing them the difference in movement.

For example, one girl can be the earth, and a boy is the moon. They hold hands in the middle of the room. As the "earth" turns slowly in place, the moon must circle around her, always facing the earth as he goes. The relationship to the sun can be demonstrated, as a third child takes the central position, and earth, with her partner moon going around her, revolve around the sun.

Sixth-graders are fascinated by the news of satellites that have been placed in orbit. They often come to school with information about the name and size of the latest satellite, and the shape of its orbit. This can be demonstrated to the rest of the class by asking one of the well-informed children to show in movement the shape of the satellites' orbit, and its relationship to other bodies in space.

The order of the planets revolving about the sun can be similarly demonstrated. What we know about various planets, their speed, the direction they face, can be acted out. Signs held by each child can represent the nature of the planet's surface or can tell other facts about it that have been discovered.

These demonstrations in movements clarify concepts for children and make difficult ideas easier to understand. In addition, just getting children out of their seats and moving increases their interest and encourages lively participation. Any one of these demonstrations can also grow and develop form so that it becomes an aesthetic experience. Science in the elementary school need not be pure logic and fact, but can deal with an emotional reaction to the wonder of our world as well.

Beauty in Nature

Why does the turtle draw up in its shell? What feeling does a moth suggest as it opens its wings for the first time?" Answering these questions involves discovery of scientific information but also deals with feeling tones and qualities. The answers can be related to the children's own experiences, so that they are no longer simply showing how a turtle pulls in, or how a moth opens out, but are expressing emotional qualities in movement.

Science study need not always be cold and factual. The beauty of the world of nature should not be ignored. Our concern for proofs and reasons should not cause us to teach science in terms of reason alone. Collections of facts do not fully account for nature as we find it nor for man's emotional response to nature. Children are curious about why things are, but they are also sensitive to the quality of their surroundings and to the effect on themselves. They want to know what makes fog, but they also feel the quiet mystery of fog.

Art expression need not be divorced from scientific learning in the school curriculum. When young children pretend that they are flowers growing out of the ground, the uplifted feeling that comes as the heads come up and the arms reach out is beautiful to watch. A suggestion to "keep shoulders down, and make necks long" helps to increase this uplifted feeling.

Flowers have different qualities, and children are quick to sense this. A gay daisy is very different from a delicate columbine. After a walk in the woods, it is fun to make dances about the various flowers that were seen.

Trees are different, too. The strong oak, the flowing willow, the outspread elm, the young sapling—all can be portrayed in movement. Interpretation through using their own bodies makes children aware of these differences.

Seeds are scattered in many ways. Maple "polly-noses" spiral down as they fall from the trees. Milkweed pops open, and then each little seed acts like a parachute and floats gently to the ground. The prickly burdock is carried along on our clothing as we walk through a field. Movement studies can be done for all these. Questions such as "How does that seed fall? Show me, Ellen!" and "Tom, how did that prickly burdock seed you found make you feel?" set the children off into imaginative movement exploration that can have exciting results.

These are short improvisations that may take a minute of class time, but they add to the liveliness of the discussion. Longer movement studies can be planned around themes like the pollination of flowers or the change of the seasons. The class can be divided into groups, each doing a section of the story in movement. With pollination as a theme, some children might represent the flowers, others might be insects. Even separate parts of the flower might be portrayed by a group studying flower parts. After pollination by the insect, they might dramatize the withering of the petals, the growth of the pistil, and the formation of the fruit.

A second-grade class finished a unit on the four seasons and decided to dramatize what they had learned. The class was divided into four groups, each representing one of the seasons. Each group presented a lovely dance to the rest of the class illustrating its season.

In the fall group, Tony was a tree, while others grouped around him were leaves that fell from its branches. Mark, representing the wind, swerved around the tree, causing a few of the leaves to fall at a time. The action of the leaves rolling along the ground as the wind blew them was also portrayed. Patty and Mike were people who raked the leaves into a pile. They lighted an imaginary match, and the pile of leaves began to burn. Fire was represented by sharp staccato movements of the arms as the children clustered close in a group. As the flames grew larger, one or two of them jumped up, and then crouched down in their original positions as others leaped. Some drifted off from the group, as the movement of the flames died down. They were the smoke! The children had selected a record of Stravinsky's "Firebird" music, and they fitted their action to it well.

The winter group chose a poem about a snowman to move to. As Perry read the poem, Heidi and Morri played in the snow, building a snowman. Tom, as the snowman, began to grow bigger as they worked at making him. Finally the snowman came alive and hopped around, playing with the children. They decided to take him home with them, but when they did he melted into a puddle near the stove.

The spring group were flowers that grew out of the ground. Barbara was a child who planted and cared for them. Ian was the sun who moved with big rounded form across the sky. Susan was the rain that dropped gently down upon the ground. The children made some lovely sound effects with the rhythm instruments to accompany their movements. Masks were made of construction and crêpe paper to represent the faces of the flowers.

The summer group showed various fruits and vegetables being harvested. Movements representing climbing trees, picking apples, digging up potatoes, driving a tractor, and carrying heavy baskets were used in an interesting combination of patterns.

Thus, for these second-graders, a science unit became an aesthetic experience. Dramatization made the ideas "come alive," while the different feelings associated with the seasons became an integral part of the study. Educators generally now believe that the "affective domain," which deals with feelings, is as important as the "cognitive domain," which deals with thinking. Appreciation of the beauty in nature can be instilled through movement experiences related to science topics.

6 ཀྭ
Creative Movement and Individual Differences

As educators, we are not concerned solely with what the child achieves in school; we are interested in the kind of person he or she will become. Today, when so many people work at routine jobs, when housing developments and mass production have given so much uniformity to life, some form of personal expression is a necessity. It provides the sense of uniqueness that gives unity and meaning to life. Creative movement can be important in contributing to the development of personality. In other art media, techniques and materials may be needed, but for dance children need only their own bodies, and the freedom to use them expressively.

The classroom teacher need not be a psychologist to be able to sense the contributions to personality growth inherent in situations involving creative movement in the classroom. Different children respond in various ways.

Overcoming Self-consciousness

Robbin is a first-grader who barely speaks above a whisper. She never volunteers for any activity. She seems happiest during rhythms sessions, when the children are allowed to skip, run, and gallop around the room. Even then, however, her movements are restrained and self-conscious. Sometimes when the children are all swinging freely or skipping in a circle, she seems more relaxed. The class had talked about "acting out" some fairy tales. Everyone had favorites to suggest. One day the children were Cinderellas and Princes. Another day they were Papa, Mama, and Baby Bears.

Robbin came quietly to the teacher's desk one morning. "Would it be too sad to do 'The Little Match Girl'?" she asked. Her mother had read the Andersen fairy tale to her the night before.

"Sad things are sometimes beautiful, too," the teacher told her.

It was hard for Robbin to get started. The teacher helped. She described the way the Match Girl looked, the way she was dressed. Soon Robbin was moving as the Match Girl might move. Her small, timid steps, so much a part of her, might have been made by this other child. The class listened and watched, for this was a story that was new to most of them. Then the Match Girl lit the match in which she was to see such lovely images. Robbin's face lit up, and her body unfolded. The movement was not big, but there was a change from the huddled position to the open one that started within the child. The teacher's voice went on, setting the mood, creating a rhythm with her pauses. Robbin's movement developed; she reached out; she turned. Finally she sank down quietly, and the dream was gone.

Robbin had forgotten about herself, and she blushed when the class applauded. This was a day she would remember.

Many children tend to lose self-consciousness when they become absorbed with a movement idea. The teacher and the class help. In Robbin's case, if attention had been called to her appearance, it may have broken her concentration and she would have become too aware of self. Instead the emphasis was strongly focused on the part she was playing, so that the child herself was hardly there. The children watching, who were quick to catch a feeling that was sincere, were held by it.

A child who does not want to participate should never be forced to do so. "You may watch today, Karen. Tomorrow you may have an idea you might want to act out."

The self-conscious child is very anxious to be part of what is happening. Opportunities can be provided that will make it easier for him or her. When the "prince" or "princess" needs two attendants, the shy child can be invited to be one of them. Being chosen by another member of the class gives the greatest encouragement. This may not work the first or second time, but soon it will.

Coping with Behavior Problems

Sally has emotional problems and is easily frustrated. She is afraid to try new things. She will scream and kick if she is not satisfied with her own accomplishments. Over the period of the term, the other children in the class have come to accept Sally's bad behavior. They sense from the teacher's attitude that Sally needs help and encouragement.

For a part of the term, Sally did not participate in rhythmic activities. She never volunteered to take part in a story for dramatization. She draws well, however, and has lots of imagination and feeling in her pictures. The children always admire her art work. Once she made a picture of the "Dog-fairy" who was a character in the story of "Noodle" in the reader. When the children decided to act that story out one day, they all wanted Sally to be the "Dog-fairy."

Sally not only acted and moved like the "Dog-fairy"; she told other children how to play rhythm instruments to accompany her. She took over part of the direction of the play. From a sulky girl with tantrums, she became an active participant and leader.

Of course, the sulking and the temper did not disappear. Her emotional problems are too deep-seated for any such miracles to happen. But since that day, she always participates when stories are acted out. She asks to do the "Dog-fairy" again and again, and it has become one of the favorites of the class. She has become a better member of the group, and she enjoys her relationship with others. She is beginning to feel accepted, and once this happens, her schoolwork is bound to improve.

Opportunities for Acceptance

The reinforcement that comes from working with others is an important aspect of movement studies. Children learn to recognize different abilities in their classmates. A child who moves well, one who has "good ideas" for dramatization may not be outstanding in other areas of schoolwork. Creative movement may provide the opportunity for leadership that is sorely needed.

Mark tries hard in school, but he just cannot sit still for long, and is likely to be playful when others are working. He falters with his reading, and his writing appears to be careless and sloppy. He is often scolded for misbehavior. His teacher has worked hard to get him to concentrate more, but he seems less mature than some of the other second-graders and has a shorter interest span.

But Mark moves expressively. He makes noises as he goes and has the uninhibited feel for combining sound and movement often exhibited by a younger child. His "steam-shovel" is so realistic in terms of both sound and movement that one almost expects a piece of the floor to come up as his arms reach like claws toward it! Children always choose him to be the airplane or the engine of the train. His "seagull" flying over the ocean is beautiful to watch. He swoops down and curves, and the gull sounds that accompany his movements accent the changes in direction. He loves the recognition the class gives him after such a performance.

Improving Coordination

The "good student" does not always relate well to the group. Such children may be excellent readers who spend all their time at passive activities. They cannot keep up with others on the playground. They have not had enough experience with large muscle activity, and are awkward and clumsy.

Steven is such a boy. His coordination is poor, and he is the last to be chosen for teams in outdoor games. He doesn't run fast, climb well, nor catch a ball easily. Although he is the best reader in the class, he would rather be an agile athlete like Vincent. Steven tags after him and begs for attention from him. Vincent moves with sureness and grace, like a young animal.

The class was working with drums one day, when Steven got his chance. Each child was to choose a partner to work with, and Vincent chose Steven! It was a wise choice, for Steven plays the drum well. He is sensitive to changes in the rhythm of his partner who is moving, and he can count beats and accents.

Vincent and Steven worked off in a corner, while other couples scattered about trying things out by themselves. Steven was enjoying this private session with his idol. He played the drum while Vincent's movements changed from walks to skips, with occasional jumps thrown in for accent. He made suggestions to Vincent. "Now stop suddenly. That's it! After the jump!"

When the class came back to the circle to see what each couple had done, Vincent's dance was good. The rhythm of Steven's drum helped to make it so. But Steven's dance was even better. With Vincent playing the drum for him, he skipped for the first time.

Channeling Energies

Many experienced teachers may be asking, "Doesn't all this activity overstimulate the children? Doesn't it cause discipline problems?" To some extent it does. Children in a state of animation are often more difficult to control than those that are dull and unresponsive. But when they are oriented toward a goal, their energies can be confined toward the attainment of their ends. When they are beginning to work out an idea, their voices may build to a crescendo, and they may jump around excitedly. But as the work period progresses, they control their enthusiasm in order to formulate their ideas and make them clear to others. They wait their turn to show what they have done. The teacher stresses the importance of being "good audience." They must not interrupt when someone is performing. They must concentrate on what is happening, and only at the end may they offer constructive suggestions. When a class watches a child or group performing, they are extremely attentive. A class watching a "dance" or a "play" maintains order without direction from the teacher. The narrator or the leader "runs the show." Others control their excitement, because they want to be sure that they will have a turn, too.

To children with excess energy, creative movement may provide a necessary release that makes them easier to deal with for the rest of the day. It is true that such children may become "wild" while moving about the room. They might throw themselves about, bumping and pushing others, and acting silly. This may be self-consciousness too. Children behaving in this way may be asked to sit down. They won't like this and will try harder next time to keep their energies under control so as not to disrupt the group activity.

For example, Richard often has to be restrained in this way during class. But there are times when he can throw himself into movement with as much abandon as he likes, and if he does not interfere with others, the group and the teacher will welcome his display of energy!

On this day the class is doing animal movements. They have taken an imaginary trip to the zoo. They are bears, lumbering along with heavy steps, arms swinging. They are seals lying on their stomachs with arched backs. They are monkeys, doing all kinds of stunts.

Richard is participating so actively that it is difficult to believe he is listening, as the teacher says, "Now we are tigers. Think of how they use their paws to feel the ground. Think about their backs, how their spines seem to wave!"

And there is Richard! He is not a tiger pacing a cage in a zoo—he is a wildcat in a jungle! His spine is liquid. He crouches and springs. His head moves out from his neck in waving motion. It goes to one side, and his arm circles over it, as a cat uses his paw to stroke himself. He is wild. But he is definitely feline!

Never could a teacher have taught such a movement to a child! It is exciting, and the whole class stops to watch it. It is good for him to know that sometimes this wild activity is not wrong. Having released his energy in a constructive and imaginative way, he was well-behaved for the rest of the day.

Developing the Gifted Child

Almost all children love to move freely, and most of them can, at some time, get expression and feeling into their movement. Some, however, are more sensitive than others. They can catch a quality in their movement. Their whole bodies are expressive, and they seem to move as a harmonious whole. We say that such children are "graceful," or that they possess "talent."

Julia began to show special ability to dance when she was in nursery school. She could catch the quality of a color, or the feel of the music, in her movements. She could be "Peter" or she could be the "Wolf" with equal ease. She created dances from all sorts of inspiration, but her dance was never quite the same when she did it again. It was always a joy to watch her. She was absorbed and seemed carried away as she moved. Now a young woman, Julia has continued to study and has had the opportunity to tour with a concert dance company. She will probably have a successful career in dance. Her early exposure to creative movement in her nursery school affected her whole life. She was encouraged to develop her sensitive responses to an artistic level.

Youngsters with artistic talent can be discovered when they have the opportunity to move creatively in school. Sometimes that talent, or sensitivity, finds expression in some other medium.

Movement frees the child for expression in other forms and is good foundation for the other art experiences. The ability to project feelings through bodily movements is needed by the actor. Freedom of movement and sensitivity is needed by the painter. Rhythmic training and a sense of phrasing is invaluable to the musician and the poet. The feeling for three-dimensional space that the dancer gets is useful in sculpture. A class that has been exposed to creative movement is more responsive to all other art forms. Art and music specialists who visit such a class once a week often remark about this. One never knows what talents might flourish in later life that were nourished in their early stages through exploration in movement.

7
Conclusion

Creative movement can be a way of exploring familiar areas of the curriculum. It has not been presented here as another subject to be studied. It is hoped that using movement exploration in the classroom will give another dimension to concepts already part of the program. Children will learn more than simply facts and their logical relationships; they will develop feelings and insights about what they have studied. Through movement, they will be exploring, not only with their eyes and ears, but with their kinesthetic sense, as well.

Creative movement is a way of working, and any teacher who creates an accepting atmosphere in the classroom can use this method. In this atmosphere, children feel free to be themselves, to share ideas and experiences with other children and with their teacher. The teacher contributes to the group and takes from it. This kind of teacher is involved in the class as a part of an alive and feeling organism.

Many teachers already work with their pupils in this manner. They may not have done movement studies, but the planning of a mural or the suggestions for organizing a research topic often involve the same kind of leadership, the same teaching techniques. For these teachers, exploring movement will feel comfortable and familiar when they try it.

Other teachers, who may be less familiar with a class situation that involves close interaction between teacher and pupils, may perhaps be aided by this advice. The whole secret is to relax and be yourself! If you respond to children naturally and unaffectedly, they will sense your sincerity and will be willing to go along with you. If they see your genuine interest in a new idea, they will be interested, too. You might even tell your class that you have read of something that might be fun to try.

You don't have to be a dancer or have had training in movement. Given the opportunity, the children will move in various ways to express their ideas. You can move about with them, or you can simply stand aside and watch. Your voice alone can guide them, and your watchful eye can detect movements that have quality and meaning. You will find that soon you too will become involved, and you will be enjoying it as much as the children.

It is hoped that some of the suggestions made in this book will be helpful in getting you started. The enthusiastic response you get from your pupils, their absorption and their imaginative ideas in movement will be more convincing than anything I can say!

Appendix A
Recommended Reading
for Teachers

Cherry, Clare. *Creative Movement for the Developing Child*. Palo Alto, Calif.: Fearon, 1968.

Dimonstein, Geraldine. *Children Dance in the Classroom*. New York: Macmillan, 1971.

Flinchum, Betty. *Motor Development in Early Childhood: A Guide for Movement Education for Six Year Olds*. St. Louis, Mo.: C. V. Mosby, 1975.

Gerhardt, Lydia. *Moving and Knowing: The Young Child Orients Himself in Space*. Englewood Cliffs, N.J.: Prentice-Hall, 1973.

Linderman, Earl W., and Donald W. Herberholz. *Developing Artistic and Perceptual Awareness: Art Practice in the Elementary Classroom*. 3rd ed. Dubuque, Iowa: W. C. Brown, 1974.

Lowenfeld, Viktor, and Lambert W. Brittain. *Creative and Mental Growth*. 6th ed. New York: Macmillan, 1975.

Mettler, Barbara. *Creative Dance in Kindergarten*. Tuscon, Ariz.: Mettler Studios, 1976.

Murray, Ruth. *Dance in Elementary Education*. New York: Harper and Row, 1953.

Sheehy, Emma. *Children Discover Music and Dance*. New York: Teachers College Press, 1974.

Stecher, Miriam B., Hugh McElleny, and Marion Greenwood. *Music and Movement Improvisation*. A Theshold Book. New York: Macmillan, 1971.

Wheeler, Lawrence, and Lois Raebeck. *Orff and Kodaly Adapted for the Elementary School*. Dubuque, Iowa: W. C. Brown, 1973.

Appendix B
Stories and Poems to Dramatize

Stories Emphasizing Characterization Through Dialogue

The following stories are listed alphabetically by title.

A *Special Trade*, by Sally Wittman. New York: Harper and Row, 1978. Bartholomew, an old man, and Neily, a little girl, go for walks together, and Bartholomew teaches Neily many things. Then when Bartholomew grows very old and is confined to a wheel chair, Neily takes him out and does things for him.

Are You My Mother? by P. D. Eastman. Random House Beginners Book. New York: Random House, 1960. A baby bird falls out of a nest and asks various animals, "Are you my mother?" He is reunited with Mama Bird at the end. First graders can read this and plan the action themselves.

Ask Mr. Bear, by Marjorie Flack. New York: Macmillan, 1971. A little boy wants to know what to give his mother for her birthday; he asks a hen, a goose, a goat, a sheep, and a cow to offer something. They respond in characteristic ways, but it isn't until Mr. Bear suggests a bear-hug that the situation is resolved satisfactorily. The story, as written, is practically in dramatic form and is fine material for the nursery-kindergarten-age group.

"Billy Goats Gruff," in *I Know a Story*. Wonder Story Books. New York: Harper and Row, 1976. As Little Billy Goat Gruff, Big Billy Goat Gruff, and Great Big Billy Goat Gruff try to cross the bridge to get to the grass on the hillside, the Ugly Troll threatens to gobble them up. The children enjoy portraying the different-sized goats both in walk and in size of voice. The Ugly Troll may hide behind a desk, and as he crouches there, his body, his face, and his voice should show his ugliness.

"Chicken Little," in *Once Upon a Time*. Wonder Story Books. New York: Harper and Row, 1976. Chicken Little believes that the sky is falling, and he tells Henny Penny, Turkey Lurkey, Ducky Lucky, Goosey Loosey, and Foxy Loxy. The repetitions in this story make it easy to dramatize.

Drummer Hoff, translated by Barbara Emberley. Englewood Cliffs, N.J.: Prentice-Hall, 1967. This is a rhyming book about firing a cannon. There is repetition of dialogue, and the action holds the interest of children.

Monster Mary Mischief Maker, by Kazuko Taniguchi. New York: McGraw-Hill, 1976. This is a story about Monster Whirlwind, Monster Starshine, Monster Sweetflower, and Monster Mary. Monster Whirlwind blows new clouds into the sky every day. Monster Starshine cuts out bright stars to light the sky at night. Monster Sweetflower paints colors on flowers, but Monster Mary does nothing but get into mischief. This is the story of how Monster Mary finds a place for herself and earns the name Monster Mary Lovingheart.

Pancakes for Breakfast, by Tomie De Paola. New York: Harcourt Brace Jovanovich, 1978. This is a high-interest, low-readability book. The story is about an old woman who wants pancakes for breakfast, but everything that can possibly go wrong happens.

"Possum was Fooled," by Shirley Patterson, in *Daisy Days*. Basics in Reading. Palo Alto, Calif.: Scott, Foresman, 1978. Possum, Racoon, and Woodpecker try to straighten out a snake only to discover it is his old skin they have found.

Really Rosie: A Musical Play, by Maurice Sendak. New York: Harper and Row, 1963. Rosie is a star, but no one believes her. She proves herself by directing several short plays. Music and lyrics are included.

"Sun and Wind" (Aesop fable), in *I Know a Story*. Wonder Story Books. New York: Harper and Row, 1976. The Sun and the Wind try to get the man on the road to take off his coat. The Wind blows hard, but huffing and puffing do no good. The Sun smiles and the day turns warm. The man takes off his coat.

"The Boy and the Goat" (Swedish folk tale), in *Once Upon A Time*.
Wonder Story Books. New York: Harper and Row, 1976. A boy has
three goats who get into the garden. A rabbit, a fox, and a wolf try to get
the goats out of the garden, but only a bee succeeds.

"The Peter Rabbit Play," in *Together We Go*. Bookmark Reading Series.
New York: Harcourt, Brace and World. 1970. Jeff gets to play Peter
Rabbit in the school play. The other children play parts of Mr. McGre-
gor, Mother Rabbit, and the other rabbits.

"The Three Bears," in *I Know a Story*. Wonder Story Books. New York:
Harper and Row, 1976. This is a favorite for acting out with young
children. Even three-year-olds can remember the lines, and can make
their voices fit the three sizes of the bears.

The Zoo in My Garden, by Chiyoko Nakatani. New York: T. Y. Crowell,
1970. A young boy describes the many animals that can be found in his
garden. Each animal can be demonstrated in movement.

Will Spring Be Early? Will Spring Be Late? by Crockett Johnson. New
York: T. Y. Crowell, 1960. A goundhog causes confusion in the animal
world when he predicts spring too soon.

Stories Emphasizing the Activity of Characters

The following stories are listed alphabetically by title.

A Wild Goose Chase, by Roy Toothaker. Englewood Cliffs, N.J.: Prentice-Hall, 1975. A boy watches a goose chase an animal that is chasing
another animal that is chasing another animal. In the end, the boy
catches the goose. A "tag" or "leap frog" might grow out of this.

Caps for Sale, adapted by Esphyr Slobodkina. New York: School Book
Service, 1976. Some monkeys steal a peddler's caps. They play tricks
with them and refuse to return them until the peddler gets a bright
idea. By throwing his own cap upon the ground, he gets the monkeys to
imitate him and to relinquish the caps. The important part of this story
is in the activity. Enlarged pantomime can lend itself to some good
comic dance.

Gobble, Growl, Grunt, by Peter Spier. Garden City, N.Y.: Doubleday,
1971. This is a beautifully illustrated book with six hundred pictures of

animals and the sounds that they make. Acting out the animals and making the sounds might develop into a guessing game.

"Gustav Green," by Ann Devendorf, in *Daisy Days*. Basics in Reading. Palo Alto, Calif.: Scott, Foresman, 1978. Gustav Green is a grasshopper who cannot hop. His cousins try to show him but to no avail. He continues walking but then develops a "step-hop" leading to a skip, and is called a "grass-skipper."

Hansel and Gretel, by the Grimm Brothers. New York: Golden Press, Western Publishing, 1976. The activities of Hansel and Gretel as they find themselves lost in the woods, discover the candy house, and experience fear of the witch can be portrayed through movement, while dialogue can be kept to the minimum. There is a good opportunity for sensing emotional qualities in this well-loved story.

Jack and the Beanstalk, as told by Stella W. Nathan. New York: Golden Press, Western Publishing, 1976. The activities of planting the seeds, climbing the beanstalk, and being chased by the Giant are essential features of the story. The difference in Jack's light steps and the Giant's heavy ones offers an interesting rhythmic contrast that the teacher might emphasize on the drum and that adds to the characterization.

Journey to the Moon, by Erich Fuchs. A Seymour Lawrence Book. New York: Delacorte Press, 1970. This is a picture book that depicts space journey. Many activities can be acted out.

Push-Pull, Empty-Full, by Tana Hobin. New York: Macmillan, 1976. A picture book of opposites. One word to a page. Each can be acted out.

The Elves and the Shoemaker, by the Grimm Brothers. New York: School Book Service, 1977. The activity of the elves, the surprise of the shoemaker and his wife, all make interesting dramatization.

The Hurdy-Gurdy Man, by Margery Bianco. New York: Gregg, 1980. A hurdy-gurdy man brings gaiety to an orderly town where people have forgotten how to play. The three tunes of the hurdy-gurdy grow in intensity and wildness. Records could supply real music at this point, and suitable dances could be devised to carry the storyline.

The Little Engine That Could, by Watty Piper. New York: School Book Service, 1979. A farmer wants to get an engine to carry his bags of wheat over the mountain. Each engine has a reason why it cannot help until a squeaky old engine makes the final effort. All of the children can form a line and make a train, as they say, "I think I can—I think I can" to accompany their movements.

Thruway, by Anne and Harlowe Rockell. New York: Macmillan, 1972. This is a story about traveling on a thruway to get where we are going. It is about going over bridges, going faster and slower, squeezing onto one lane, and passing other cars. It is easy to visualize the story with children instead of cars doing the action.

Stories Emphasizing Mood

The following stories are listed alphabetically by title.

Autumn Harvest, by Alvin Tresselt. New York: Lothrop, Lee and Shepard, 1960. Descriptions of autumn scenes and events are given in poetic prose, with images drawn that stimulate imagination. Some of the activities described could be dramatized or an interpretation might be given to one of the images. The illustrations help to convey the mood to be interpreted.

Good Night, by Elizabeth Coatsworth. New York: Macmillan, 1972. This story is about what a star sees. It can see a mother and a baby, a mare and a colt, a dog and her puppies, and a cat family. Then the child goes to bed, and the star follows him as he goes to sleep. This would be effective read to background music as the children act it out in pantomime.

How I Feel, by June Behrens. Chicago: Childrens' Press, 1973. This is a good opportunity for the children to express different feelings. Some examples from the book are "proud," "sad," and "lonesome." Suitable music might be played on a record as the children portray the various feelings.

Parsley, by Ludwig Bemelmans. New York: Harper and Row, 1955. This is a story of a friendship between an old pine tree and an old stag known as "Parsley." The tree saves the stag from a hunter. The descriptions of the tree in different seasons, the movement of the wind, and the actions of the stag and the hunters lend themselves to dance interpretation.

Talking Without Words, by Marie Hall Ets. New York: Viking Press, 1968. This book presents a creative way to develop the concept of nonverbal communication. This is accomplished by showing the daily activities of animals and people. Some examples are shrugging shoulders, rubbing tummy, putting a finger over lips, and waving.

The Country Noisy Book, by Margaret Wise Brown. New York: Harper and Row, 1976. The sounds and feelings of the country are described, as heard through the ears of a little dog, Muffin. All of the Noisy Books emphasize sensory impressions and lend themselves to movement interpretation by young children.

The Day We Saw the Sun Come Up, by Alice E. Goudey. New York: Scribner's, 1961. The awe and wonder of the world and the sun are described, as seen through children's eyes. Sections that deal with stealing through the grass in early morning dew, playing with their shadows, and other movements can be interpreted, and effort can be made to catch the quality of awe and wonder in the book.

The Tale of the Yellow Triangle, by Gustaf Sobin. New York: Braziller, 1973. This is a beautifully written and illustrated book about moods. It is about the change and the different forms our minds and our bodies go through to achieve change. There are many movement and drama activities suggested in the story plus invaluable lessons for children to learn and to experience.

What Did You Leave Behind? by Alvin Tresselt. New York: Lothrop, Lee and Shepard. 1978. This book is about going to different places, the different things we bring home (example: sand from the beach), and what we leave behind (example: the shore breeze, the salt taste of the water). The question is raised as to whether we really leave these things behind or if we take them along in our memories.

Where the Wild Things Are, by Maurice Sendak. New York: Harper and Row, 1963. This is a favorite with children who love to see the scary illustrations of "the wild things." Monsters and dragons can be acted out in movement, with background music such as *Dance Macabre*. This is especially good at Halloween time.

Poetry

All the poems mentioned in the text and many others that would be good for movement interpretation may be found in the following collections:

Aldis, Dorothy. *All Together*. New York: Putnam, 1952.

Arbuthnot, May Hill. *The Arbuthnot Anthology of Children's Literature*. 4th ed. New York: Lothrop, Lee and Shepard, 1976.

Browning, Robert. *The Pied Piper of Hamelin*. Illustrated by Kate Greenway. London: Frederick Warne, 1889.

Coatsworth, Elizabeth. *Poems*. New York: Macmillan, 1958.

Lear, Edward. *Complete Nonsense Book*. New York: Dover, 1951.

Lindsay, Vachel. *Johnny Appleseed and Other Poems*. Greenport, N.Y.: Harmony & Co., 1981.

Milne, A. A. *The World of Christopher Robin*. New York: Dutton, 1958.

Richards, Laura E. *Tirra-Lirra*. Boston: Little, Brown, 1955.

Stevenson, Robert Louis. *A Child's Garden of Verses*. New York: Random House, 1978.

Teachers' Guides

Additional suggestions for teachers may be found in the annotated bibliographies in the following books:

Kase, C. Robert. *Stories for Creative Acting*. New York: French, 1961.

Larrick, Nancy. *A Teacher's Guide to Children's Books*. Columbus, Ohio: Charles Merrill, 1960.

McCaslin, Nellie. *Creative Dramatics in the Classroom*. New York: David McKay, 1974.

Ward, Winifred, ed. *Stories to Dramatize*. Anchorage: Children's Theatre Press, 1952.

Appendix C
Selected List
of Recordings

Below is a very limited listing of recommended records for classroom use. I have not noted recording companies for each selection, since many of these have been recorded by several companies. Most of the selections listed here are available from Educational Record Sales, 157 Chambers Street, New York, N.Y. 10007, and are listed in their catalog. They may also be found in other catalogs for educational materials and in local music stores.

In addition to the following selections, many others have appeal for children and are available in schools. New action and story records are released each year by record companies. Often children like to bring these to class, and some are suitable for creative movement.

Classical Music

Whenever possible, classical selections are preferred, since exposure to fine music is both desirable and exciting for children.

Carnival of the Animals (Saint-Saens)

Children's Corner Suite (Debussy) Includes "Dr. Gradus and Parnassum," "Jimbo's Lullaby," "Serenade for the Doll," "The Snow is Dancing," "The Little Shepherd," "Golliwogg's Cakewalk," and "Suite Bergamasque" (which includes the well-known "Claire de Lune").

Dance Macabre (Saint-Saens)

For Children (Bartok) Vols. I and II: 15 Hungarian Peasant Songs,
   Roumanian Dances, "Piano Sonata," "Petite Suite," and others.

Nutcracker Suite (Tchaikovsky) Includes "March," "Spanish Dance,"
   "Arabian Dance," "Chinese Dance," "Trepak," "Dance of the Mirli-
   tons," "Waltz of the Flowers," "Dance of the Sugar Plum Fairy."

Peter and the Wolf (Prokofiev)

Sleeping Beauty (Tchaikovsky)

Sorcerer's Apprentice (Dukas)

Music for Movement

Aerobic Dancing for Kids (Glass and Hallum) Includes "Little Man from
   Mars," "Jello," "Jumping Little, Little Jerry," "Popcorn," "Four Walls
   Game," and Teachers' Guide.

Classroom Rhythm Library Includes six records, sold singly: *Classroom
   Rhythms, Animal Rhythms, Rhythms from the Land of Make-Believe,
   Interpretive Rhythms, Rhythms of Cowboys and Indians, Machine
   Rhythms*.

Creative Movement and Rhythmic Exploration Songs describe actions for
   children to work out in their own ways. Includes music for creative
   movement, mimetics, physical activities, and basic skills.

Discovery Through Movement Exploration Four areas in primary movement exploration are presented: space awareness, classroom related
   activities, ball and rope handling.

Elementary Floor Exercise Music Music selected for gymnastic stunts.
   Includes "Matchmaker," "Cabaret," "Theme from "Love Story," "It's
   Impossible," "The Look of Love," Teachers' Manual.

Fundamental Steps and Rhythms Includes music for walking, running,
   jumping, hopping, leaping, skipping, galloping, and sliding. Also
   Teachers' Manual.

Movement Fun Activities include imitating animals, swimming, throwing, jack-in-the-box, dump truck. Also Teachers' Manual.

Music for Movement Exploration Children are encouraged to move as
   they feel to the sounds they hear: "Aquarius," "Simon Says," "Alley
   Cat," "In a Persian Market," "Love is Blue."

Music for Rhythms and Dance Includes action music (for walking, running, turning, jumping, and skipping); waltz, march, and swing music; and mood music (angry, sad, funny, mysterious, lively). Second side: "The Pied Piper." May be ordered from Freda Miller Records for Dance, 131 Bayview Ave., Northport, N.Y. 11768.

Folk Music

Any folk music has a strong rhythmic beat and a simplicity easily reflected in children's movement. Some special favorites follow.

Burl Ives Sings Includes "The Little White Duck," "The Little Engine That Could," "The Gray Goose," "Buckeye Jim," "The Taylor and the Mouse," "Two Little Owls."

Ella Jenkins Record Library Includes *Early Childhood Songs, Call and Response, This is Rhythm, Rhythms of Childhood, You'll Sing a Song and I'll Sing a Song, Adventures in Rhythm, Songs and Rhythms from Near and Far,* and others. Records sold singly.

Singing Games Through Folk Dancing Six albums with representative music from different countries, becoming more intricate after an introduction through simple games including "Put Your Finger in the Air" (Guthrie), "Looby Loo," "Clap Your Hands," "Did you Ever See a Lassie?"

Musical Shows

Shows, such as the following, that feature good dancing usually contain good music for children's movement.

Carousel (Rogers and Hammerstein) Especially for the "Carousel Waltz," "Hornpipe," and ballet music.

Don't Bother Me, I Can't Cope especially for "Gotta Keep Movin'!"

Peter Pan Any verson includes music for flying and the pirates' dance.

West Side Story (Bernstein) Especially for the accompaniment for the street scene fights.

Story and Activity Records

These activity records provide a simple way for the teacher to start creative movement. They are somewhat limiting, however, as they often provide the child with too much suggestion and control the amount of time devoted to each movement idea. It is advisable that the teacher use the story and music flexibly.

All About Fall, All About Spring, All About Summer, All About Winter
   Four records, each with twelve songs related to the theme of the season. Accompanying book suggests a variety of activities.

Cinderella (Prokofiev)

Free to Be You and Me (Marlo Thomas) Songs that develop self-concept can be acted out.

Hansel and Gretel (Humperdinck)

Nursery Rhymes for Dramatic Play Includes "Little Miss Muffet," "Ride a Cock Horse," "Little Jack Horner," and others. Teachers' Manual.

Songs About My Feelings Moving the way you feel, with appropriate music to accompany activities.

Song Dramatizations for Children Includes "Tailor and the Mouse" and some new songs for dramatization.

The Pied Piper (Miller) Order from Freda Miller Records for Dance, 131 Bayview Ave., Northport, N.Y. 11768

Tubby the Tuba Music tells story of a tuba that wanted to play a melody. Each instrument of orchestra is represented by a different tune.

What Will I Be When I Grow Up? Music and songs to accompany action about being a teacher, doctor, policeman, farmer, and others.

Index

LIBRARY
COLLEGE OF ST. BENEDICT
St. Joseph Minnesota 56374